Twin Studies:

Research in Genes, Teeth and Faces

This book is available as a free fully-searchable ebook from
www.adelaide.edu.au/press

Twin Studies:

Research in Genes, Teeth and Faces

by

Grant C Townsend, Sandra K Pinkerton,
James R Rogers, Michelle R Bockmann
and Toby E Hughes

*School of Dentistry,
The University of Adelaide*

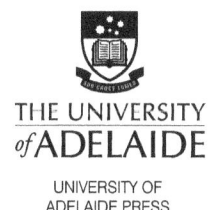

UNIVERSITY OF
ADELAIDE PRESS

Published in Adelaide by

University of Adelaide Press
The University of Adelaide
Level 14, 115 Grenfell Street
South Australia 5005
press@adelaide.edu.au
www.adelaide.edu.au/press

The University of Adelaide Press publishes externally refereed scholarly books by staff of the University of Adelaide. It aims to maximise access to the University's best research by publishing works through the internet as free downloads and for sale as high quality printed volumes.

© 2015 The authors

This work is licenced under the Creative Commons Attribution-NonCommercial-NoDerivatives 4.0 International (CC BY-NC-ND 4.0) License. To view a copy of this licence, visit http://creativecommons.org/licenses/by-nc-nd/4.0 or send a letter to Creative Commons, 444 Castro Street, Suite 900, Mountain View, California, 94041, USA. This licence allows for the copying, distribution, display and performance of this work for non-commercial purposes providing the work is clearly attributed to the copyright holders. Address all inquiries to the Director at the above address.

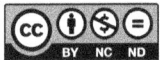

For the full Cataloguing-in-Publication data please contact the National Library of Australia: cip@nla.gov.au

ISBN (paperback) 978-1-925261-14-1
ISBN (ebook) 978-1-925261-15-8

Editor: Rebecca Burton
Editorial Support: Julia Keller
Book design: Midland Typesetters Pty Ltd
Cover design: Emma Spoehr
Cover images: Courtesy of the authors

FOREWORD

This book presents a unique account of a comprehensive research program on the genetics of teeth and faces, carried out over three decades at the School of Dentistry within the University of Adelaide by Professor Grant Townsend and colleagues. It is unique in several senses, firstly in that perhaps no other centre in the world has carried out such a long-term and wide-ranging program on so many facets of dentistry and craniofacial biology. But it is also unique in the sense that I know of no other academic endeavour that has so thoroughly documented its own history and intellectual progression, including the description not just of the main projects but also the smaller side-projects and all the people, including other researchers and students, who carried them out. Thus the book is not just a heartfelt 'thank you' to all the twins and their families who took part in these studies over the decades, but also a valuable scientific and photographic record of the research projects, their planning, execution and findings.

I am privileged to have played some small part in this research program in introducing Grant and his team to structural equation modelling methods for analysis of twin data. The great attraction for me was (and still is) not only the inherent interest in the dentition, but that the measurements are so very reliable and the traits are so heritable. This is in contrast to my other domain of interest, human behaviour, where, for many traits, measurement is often quite unreliable and heritabilities are modest. Another appealing feature of the dentition is that the same basic structure of eight teeth is replicated four times — left and right sides, on both upper and lower jaws. This provides very rich opportunities for statistical modelling, and Grant and I spent many hours, days, weeks fitting what I think are rather elegant models to explain the genetics of tooth size.

Another inherently appealing aspect of this research is that its research subjects are normal identical (monozygotic) and non-identical (dizygotic) twins growing up together in normal Australian households. In fact, the classical twin method — the comparison of the similarity of the two types of twins — is the most powerful design we have in humans to estimate the relative influence of genes and environment on any trait one cares to measure. Twins occur more or less at random throughout society, so carrying out a project of this size and duration represents quite a large-scale societal engagement with science and its methods, to the benefit of all parties — the twins find out a lot about their teeth and other aspects of their health and, most importantly for same-sex pairs (two-thirds of all twins), whether, from powerful objective blood tests, they are identical or non-identical. The researchers obtain beautiful and powerful data from willing, interested — and interesting — volunteer subjects.

Despite its simplicity and widespread use (and perhaps because some people do not like the answers it gives), the classical twin design has been subject to repeated criticism as producing estimates of heritability (genetic influence) biased upwards from their true values, mainly on the grounds that identical (monozygotic — MZ) twins are 'freakish' or 'atypical' and therefore cannot tell us anything about 'normal' individuals. However, Peter Visscher and colleagues have developed a clever new method (called Genome-Wide Complex Trait Analysis, or GCTA) for estimating heritability in a completely different way, making use of large-scale molecular genotyping on thousands of unrelated individuals. Initial estimates using GCTA did indeed suggest that twin heritabilities were somewhat inflated, but as the analyses have become more sophisticated it is gradually emerging that, for most traits, there is a high degree of consistency between the 'molecular heritability' and the twin heritability. This can be seen as a great endorsement of the twin method (and a comfort to twin researchers) and comes at a particularly auspicious time for the launch of the current book!

Like any good science, the work described in these chapters raises more questions than it answers. In particular, knowing that the dentition is so strongly genetically influenced whets the appetite to know what the particular genes are that are involved, and how they act. Only ten years ago, it seemed impossible to answer such a question but in 2005 the first successful genome-wide association study (GWAS) was published, in which hundreds of thousands of genetic markers (SNPs) are typed on large samples of cases and controls. That study found an entirely new and unsuspected gene influencing risk of age-related macular degeneration, the most common cause of blindness in old people. Since that time there have been thousands of GWAS studies published on hundreds of different biomedical traits and diseases, and new genes have been found for many of them, elucidating the biological processes shaping complex traits; for example, over 700 genes have been identified influencing

Foreword

human height. In this book Grant Townsend and his colleagues convince us of the huge importance of genes in shaping teeth, when they emerge, how big they are, how susceptible they are to decay and other dental anomalies. Surely now is the time to exploit the powerful new molecular technologies becoming available and take our understanding of the mouth, and all that is therein, to a new detailed level!

Nick Martin
Queensland Institute of Medical Research
Brisbane

PREFACE

This volume is about an ongoing long-term research initiative led by researchers from the School of Dentistry at the University of Adelaide. The aim of this book is to provide an overview of our studies of the teeth and faces of Australian twins and their families — studies that have extended over more than thirty years. Rather than providing detailed accounts of the methodologies and results of each of the individual research projects, we have provided general descriptions of the approaches that have been adopted, and have emphasised some of our key findings.

The book is aimed primarily at the participants of our studies — over 1200 pairs of twins and more than 2000 of their family members — as well as other families of twins who may be interested in being involved in future research projects. A common question asked by participants over the years has been, 'What have you found?' We now hope that these generous people, without whom our studies would have been impossible, will enjoy reading about our research in a single volume, rather than having to go through a large number of more focused, technical articles published in various journals.

The book provides some historical perspectives of studies of twins, including those involving teeth and faces. It also gives an insight into the technological and scientific changes that have occurred over the past thirty years, including various twin models that enable exploration of genetic, epigenetic and environmental contributions to variation in teeth and faces. For this reason, it should also be of interest to students planning to undertake research involving twins, as well as to researchers and academics in the fields of dentistry and craniofacial biology. We are now in the so-called 'omics' era, but the importance of twin studies has not diminished, as some had predicted it would. Rather, studies of twins and their families have become even more relevant to understanding how genetic, epigenetic and environmental factors contribute to observed variation in health and disease.

One of the features of the studies described in this book is that several of them incorporate a longitudinal design, meaning that the twins were examined on more than

Preface

one occasion. This has enabled questions to be asked about how genetic factors influence growth and development over time. The book also shows why an interdisciplinary approach can be so valuable, and how studies that are mainly focused on dental features can have broader implications in clarifying general biological mechanisms.

The first chapter of this book provides a 'tour of the mouth', introducing dental terms and concepts for those without a detailed knowledge of dentistry. The second chapter provides a historical account of twins and twinning, including how societies tended to view twins in the past. The contributions of some of the key figures who studied twins, including Francis Galton, are also summarised in this chapter. Chapter Three focuses on key researchers worldwide who have studied human teeth and faces using samples of twins. Three eras are identified: from the early 1920s to the 1940s; from the 1950s to the 1980s; and from the 1990s to the present.

Chapters Four, Five and Six describe the three main cohorts of twins included in our studies, as well as highlighting research questions posed, methods of analysis adopted, and some key findings. These chapters include many illustrations of participants and researchers.

The first cohort of twins included around 300 pairs of mainly teenage twins living in Adelaide, as well as their siblings. The second cohort involved over 300 pairs of young twins aged around 4 to 5 years of age from South Australia and Victoria, who were examined on three occasions, corresponding to when they had primary teeth, mixed dentitions, and then permanent teeth. Siblings of the twins and some parents were also included. The third cohort comprised over 600 pairs of twins and their families, including siblings and parents. These latter families have come from all over Australia and have carried out much of the record collection themselves initially, which involved processes including recording times of tooth emergence of their twins and collecting samples of dental plaque and cheek cells for subsequent microbiological assessment and DNA analysis. We are currently examining many of the twins in this third cohort in the clinic to determine the types of bacteria in their mouths and to record the development of any dental decay.

Chapter Seven includes a detailed summary of the published papers arising from our studies of twins, as well as theses completed by Honours and postgraduate students. We have also added a Glossary to help readers understand some of the dental and scientific terms that have been used in the book, and we have included an Appendix which provides a list of colleagues, visiting researchers, collaborators and key contributors, as well as more photographs of twins and their families participating in our studies and some of the researchers who have been involved in gathering records from the twins. Hopefully, these photographs will convey a sense of the enjoyment that both groups have experienced over the years.

Grant Townsend
Sandra Pinkerton
James Rogers
Michelle Bockmann
Toby Hughes

DEDICATION

This book is dedicated to all of the twins and their families who have participated in our ongoing studies and to the research and support staff who have made it all happen.

PHOTOGRAPHIC ACKNOWLEDGEMENTS

All photographs and illustrations in this book, unless otherwise attributed, are the property of

The Craniofacial Biology Research Unit

School of Dentistry

The University of Adelaide

All participants in the twin studies have given permission for their photographs to be used. Their names have been deleted, except for Jane and Carolyn Ferrett, our first pair of twins, who gave permission for their names to be included.

ETHICAL APPROVAL

Ethical approval has been granted for all of our studies of twins by the Human Ethics Committee of the University of Adelaide.

ACKNOWLEDGEMENTS

We wish to express our sincere thanks to the twins, triplets and their families who have agreed to participate in our studies over the past thirty years.

We also wish to acknowledge the support of the Australian NHMRC Twin Registry and the Australian Multiple Birth Association.

Support for this research has been provided by grants from the National Health and Medical Research Council (NHMRC) of Australia — including several project grants, a five-year Competing Epidemiological Grant and a grant to establish a Clinical Centre for Research Excellence (CCRE). Support was also provided by the Australian Dental Research Foundation, the Australian Dental Industry Association, the Australian Society of Orthodontics Foundation for Research and Education, the University of Adelaide — including the Centre for Oro-facial Research and Learning (CORAL) — and the Financial Markets Foundation for Children.

We want especially to acknowledge the ongoing support provided by Colgate Oral Care Australia, which has enabled us to give packs of oral health products to participating families. Thanks also to the South Australian Dental Service and staff of the Adelaide Dental Hospital for providing access to their clinical facilities and assisting with examination visits. Thanks as well to staff of the former Dental Therapy School Melbourne, on St Kilda Road, and to staff of the Royal Dental Hospital of Melbourne, the Melbourne Dental School and the Colgate Australian Clinical Dental Research Centre, Adelaide. Thanks to Christine Swann for several of the illustrations and Corinna Bennett for photography. A special thanks to Ms Karen Squires for her excellent work in helping to put this book together.

Thank you to all of the people who have helped at various stages of the research, including colleagues in Adelaide, Sydney, Canberra, Brisbane, Perth and Melbourne, postgraduate, Honours and undergraduate students, research collaborators, clinical examiners, recorders, dental assistants and clinic staff.

Without all of this support, we would not have been able to carry out our research.

CONTENTS

Foreword · v
Preface · viii
Dedication · xi
Photographic acknowledgements · xi
Ethical approval · xi
Acknowledgements · xii

Chapter One — A tour of the mouth · 1
Introduction · 1
How do our faces and teeth develop? · 3
What is the normal timing and sequence of dental development? · 7
What is the normal timing and sequence of tooth emergence? · 7
What are the main features of the primary and permanent teeth? · 10
How are the teeth arranged in the oral cavity? · 13
Tooth notation · 13
What are the main tissues that make up a tooth? · 16
How can we study dental morphology? · 18
Why is the dentition such a good model system for studying development? · 20
What are some of the common developmental anomalies affecting teeth? · 21
What are the most important diseases or problems that can affect our teeth? · 25
Is there a relationship between oral health and general health? · 27
Why might twins' teeth look the same or different? · 29
References · 34

Chapter Two — A historical perspective · 35
Introduction · 35
Mythological beginnings · 36
Twins in the theatre · 38

Twins in literature	39
Twins in science	41
The concept of nature versus nurture	46
Inheritance and Mendelian genetics	51
Twin research: a question of ethics	53
Twin research: specialisation	55
Twin research: the great steps forward	56
References	59

Chapter Three — Phases of research involving twin studies of teeth and faces — 62

Studies of twin resemblance: hereditary and environmental influences	62
Understanding genetic control over dental variation	67
Development of more sophisticated methods: path analysis, model-fitting and genetic expression	73
Studies of twins: the Adelaide Dental School	76
References	80

Chapter Four — Cohort 1: Teeth and faces of South Australian teenage twins — 87

Introduction	87
Cohort 1 (April 1983)	89
Methodology and data acquisition	90
Fitting genetic models to dental data from twins	99
Some key findings of our studies involving Cohort 1	104
References	109

Chapter Five — Cohort 2 – A longitudinal study of dental and facial development in Australian twins and their families — 113

Introduction	113
Collection of records and examination of twins	118
Cohort 2 as a longitudinal study	124
Twins in Melbourne	126
Some key findings of our studies involving Cohort 2	129
References	133

Contents

Chapter Six — Cohort 3 – Tooth emergence and oral health in Australian twins and their families **135**
Introduction											135
The vagaries of the grant funding process						141
Getting beaten to the punch								141
An exciting new collaboration								144
Developments in epigenetics								145
Next-generation sequencing								149
A new NHMRC grant									151
The future										154
Some of the key findings relating to Cohort 3						158
References										161

Chapter Seven — Publications and theses relating to the Adelaide Twin Studies **165**
1980s											165
1990s											166
2000s											168
2010 to 2015										171
Theses											175

Glossary of terms									**178**

Appendix 1										**185**

Chapter One

A TOUR OF THE MOUTH

INTRODUCTION

On 27 April 1983, identical twins Jane and Carolyn, aged 15 years, arrived at the Adelaide Dental School as the first participants in our new study of the teeth and faces of twins. The girls would have been wondering what they might be asked to do and we, as researchers, hoped that all our planning would translate into an enjoyable and scientifically valuable experience.

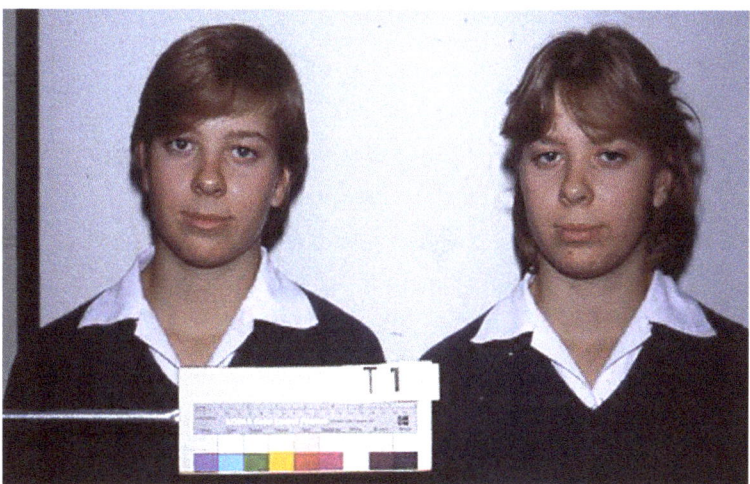

Figure 1.1
Twins 1A and 1B, Jane (right) and Carolyn Ferrett (left).

Jane and Carolyn would represent the beginning of a series of studies involving Australian twins and their families that has spanned over thirty years and is still continuing in 2015.

Over 1200 pairs of twins and over 2000 family members have participated in our studies (Hughes et al., 2013; 2014), freely giving their time to help advance knowledge about how genetic, epigenetic and environmental factors contribute to variation in the development and appearance of human teeth and faces, and to clarify further the nature of the twinning process.

Although the concept of genetic and environmental contributions to observed variation has been referred to often over the years and is familiar to most, epigenetics is a term that has only become widely used in recent times. Figure 1.2 provides a musical metaphor that emphasises how epigenetic factors influence the expression of genes to produce the variation observed in different features (referred to as phenotypes).

The aim of this opening chapter is to provide sufficient background information about the development and morphology of human teeth and faces so that, hopefully, the reader can make sense of the material presented subsequently. This chapter also introduces some relevant dental terminology that will be familiar to dental researchers but may not be so familiar to readers without a background in dentistry. Our reasons for believing that teeth and faces are so valuable for studying the roles of genetic, epigenetic and environmental factors on development in twins are also highlighted.

We commence by reviewing the main stages and processes involved in the development of teeth and faces. The way in which the teeth are arranged in the mouth and the tissues that make up teeth are also discussed. Some of the reasons why the teeth as a group (referred to as the dentition) provide such a good model system for investigating human development are provided and some of the methods that can be used to study dental morphology are described.

Although our studies of twins have often addressed basic aspects of human growth and development, our research has become increasingly more focused on oral health. We anticipate that the findings from these studies will lead, in the longer term, to improved methods of diagnosing and managing oral diseases and abnormalities. For this reason, a brief introduction to some of the more common dental anomalies has been included. The two most common dental diseases are also described: dental decay (dental caries) that may lead to toothache and loss of vitality of teeth; and gum

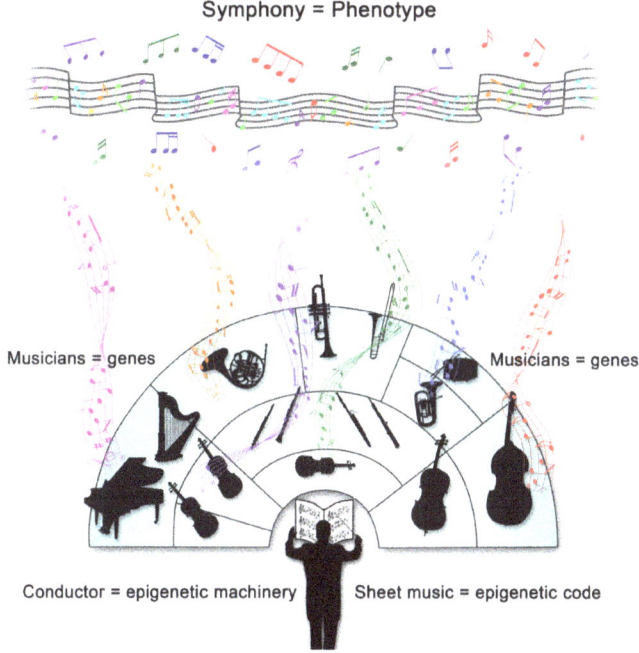

Figure 1.2
A musical metaphor for how epigenetic factors influence the expression of our genetic code to produce variation in different features. The sheet music represents the epigenetic code, the conductor represents the epigenetic machinery, the musicians represent the individual genes, and the resultant sound is equivalent to the phenotype. Reproduced with permission from the Australian Dental Journal (Williams et al., 2014).

disease (gingivitis) that may lead on to the destruction of the supporting tissues of the tooth (periodontal disease).

Recent research has provided support for links between oral health and general health, and vice versa, and this issue is also introduced in this first chapter.

How do our faces and teeth develop?

Development of our faces begins around twenty-five days in utero with the appearance of localised tissue swellings and the migration of cells, referred to as neural crest cells, into the underlying tissue. These neural crest cells are derived from the ectoderm in the embryo, one of three layers of primitive tissue along with the mesoderm and endoderm. The primitive mouth (referred to as the stomatodeum or stomodeum), is surrounded initially by the frontonasal process, maxillary and mandibular processes. The oropharyngeal membrane, which separates the primitive mouth from the pharynx, then begins to break down. This marks the establishment of a communication between the oral cavity and the rest of the gastrointestinal tract. Soon after, the nasal pits form and odontogenic (or tooth-forming) epithelium develops where the upper and lower teeth will form (Figure 1.3).

The continuous band of thickened epithelium is referred to as the dental lamina. At each of the ten places where primary teeth will usually form in both the upper and lower jaws, thickenings of the dental lamina (tooth buds) appear which go

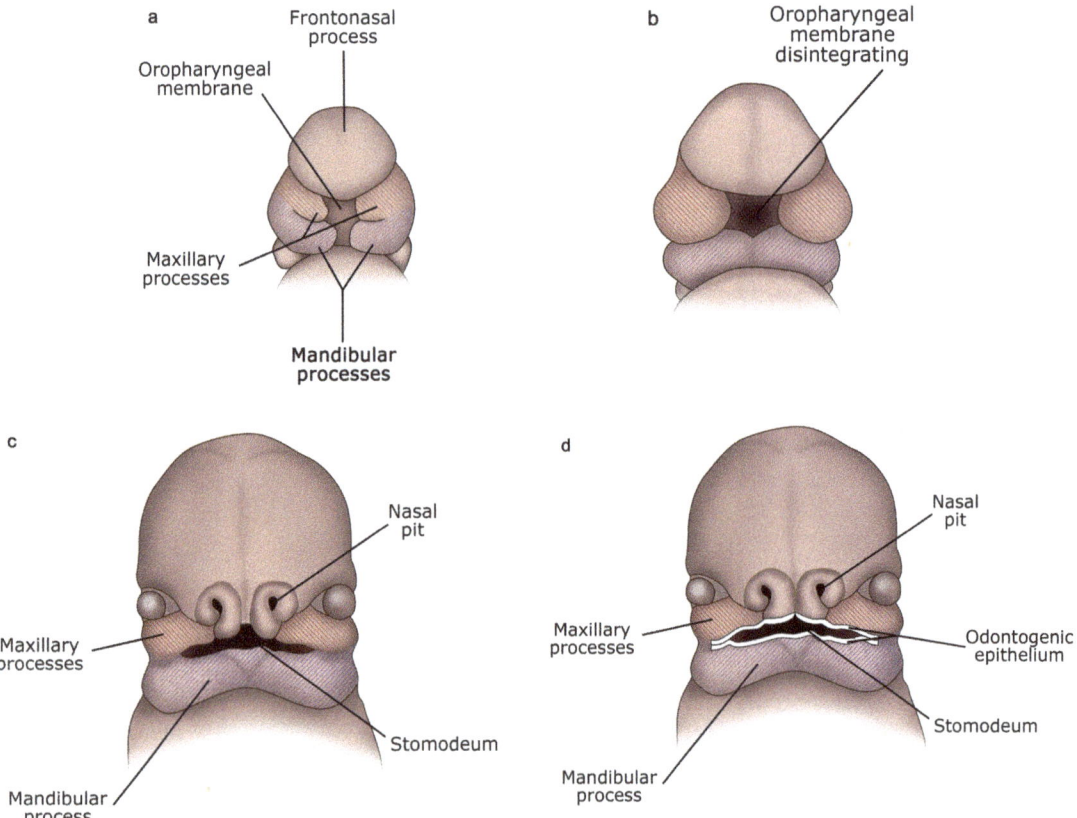

Figure 1.3
Early stages of development of the face and teeth.

on to produce structures referred to as enamel organs. An enamel organ comprises an epithelial cap that sits over a ball of condensed mesenchyme, which is referred to as the dental papilla. The enamel organ and dental papilla, with their surrounding sac, are referred to as a tooth germ (Figure 1.4).

The interactions that occur between the inner cells of the enamel organ, the so-called inner enamel epithelium, and the mesenchyme of the dental papilla into which neural crest cells migrate, are referred to as epithelial-mesenchymal interactions. These interactions, mediated by various signalling molecules and growth factors, influence folding of the inner enamel epithelium, which in turn determines the future shape of the dental crown — that is, whether the tooth will become an incisor or a molar (Figure 1.5).

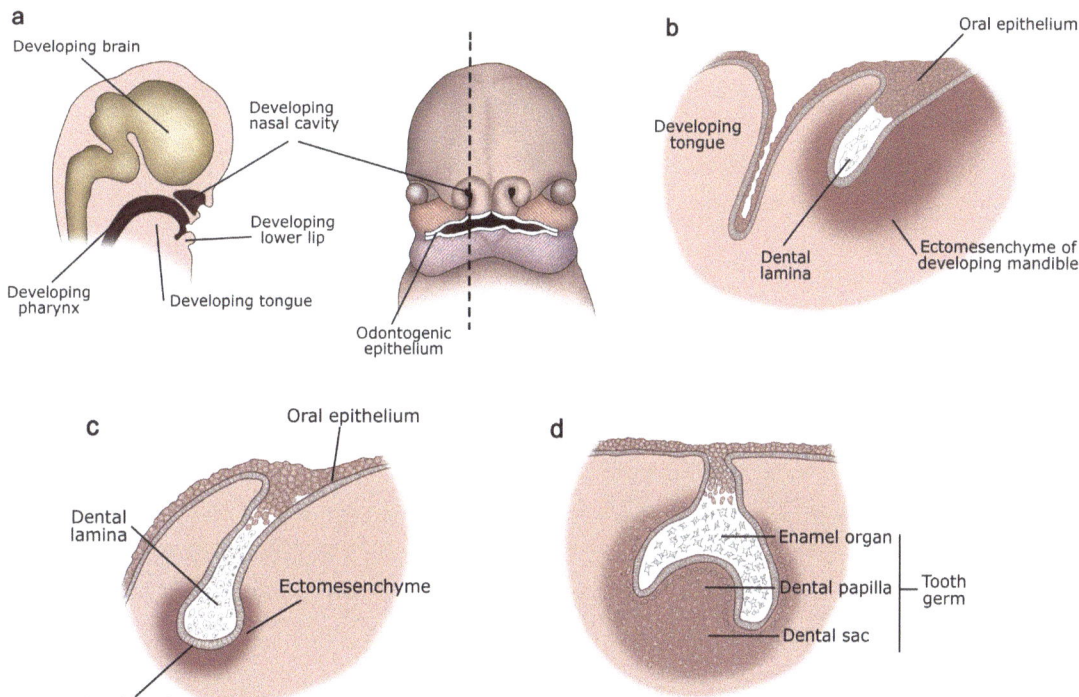

Figure 1.4
The sagittal section indicated in (a) allows the dental lamina to be visualised in (b), a tooth bud in (c), and a developing tooth germ in (d).

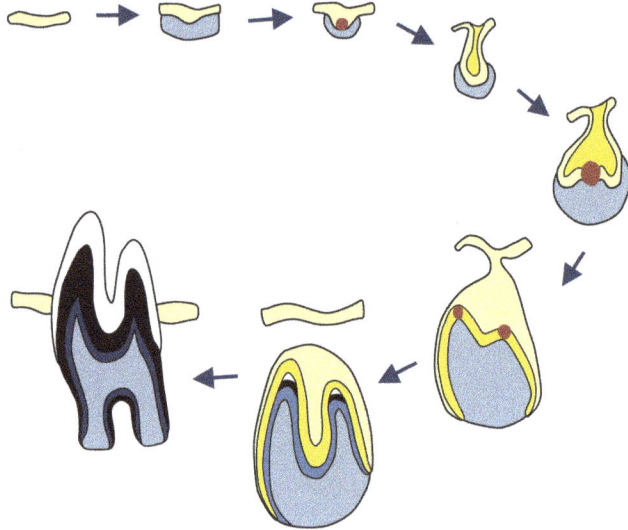

Figure 1.5
Stages of dental development, commencing with a down-growth of epithelium (yellow) towards the underlying mesenchyme (grey). This is followed by the formation of the primary enamel knot (red circle) and then the folding of the inner enamel epithelium with formation of secondary enamel knots. Enamel and dentine are laid down and the crown of the tooth is formed prior to emergence into the oral cavity.

In the past, studies focused on explaining the nature and extent of variation in fully formed teeth (so-called phenotypic variation) and then making inferences about the developmental processes that led to observed variability. However, molecular biologists have made great advances over the past decade or so in identifying the various signalling molecules that pass back and forward between epithelial and mesenchymal tissues in developing dental tissues, leading to initiation, proliferation, differentiation and morphogenesis of teeth. Furthermore, the development of modern genome-wide scanning approaches means that it is now possible to search for the specific genes that are involved in the process of dental development.

The tooth is an excellent model system for studying developmental processes in general as it can be grown in vitro, and the epithelial and mesenchymal parts can be separated and then recombined. The dentition, including all of the teeth, is also a very useful model system to study the development and arrangement of structures that show patterning and modularity in their morphology — for example, incisors, canines, premolars and molars. The arrangement of the teeth in dental arches also allows symmetrical and asymmetrical expression of features on corresponding teeth from the right and left sides to be explored.

What is the normal timing and sequence of dental development?

While the first signs of development of the primary (or deciduous) teeth are evident around four to six weeks in utero, it is not until around eighteen weeks that the crowns of these teeth begin to calcify — that is, it is not until then that enamel and dentine are laid down. By birth, all of the primary tooth crowns have usually begun to calcify, although only the regions where the tips of the cusps will be located have calcified in the primary second molars. The calcification process for the permanent dentition is usually a postnatal event, with the first molars commencing to calcify around birth and then the second and third molars starting to calcify some years later. Each tooth passes through a definite series of stages during its development, commencing with calcification of the crown followed by formation of the root(s) of the tooth. Usually the roots of teeth are about two-thirds formed when they appear in the mouth, and further root development occurs after emergence until the apex of the root is fully formed (Figure 1.6).

What is the normal timing and sequence of tooth emergence?

The primary teeth tend to emerge into the oral cavity between the ages of around 6 to 8 months and 2.5 years, although there is considerable variation in the timing and sequence. The primary lower central incisors are usually the first teeth to emerge, with the second molars being the last (Table 1.1).

Variations in the sequence of emergence are not uncommon, and we have documented some of the common variations in publications based on data derived from twins enrolled in our studies.

Each primary tooth is normally shed, or exfoliated, prior to the emergence of its permanent successor. The first permanent teeth to emerge are usually the lower central incisors around the age of 6 years, while the third molars may not emerge

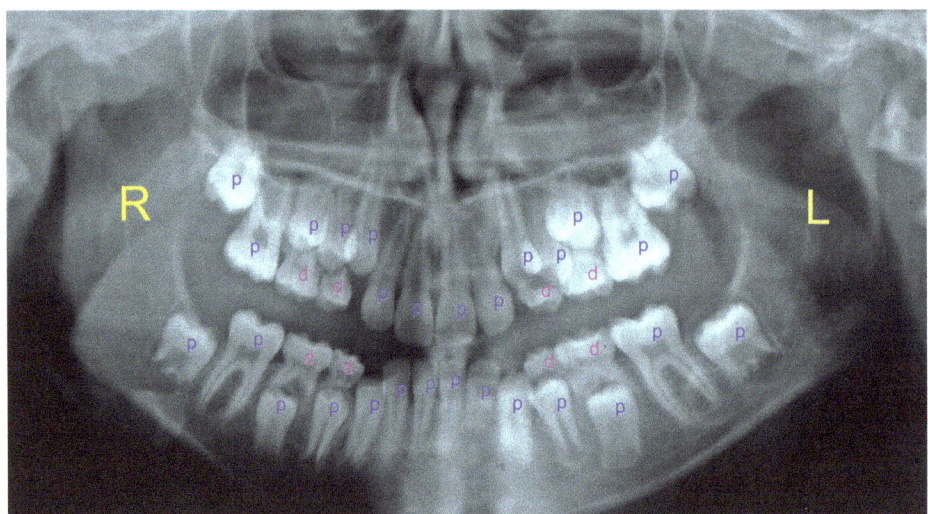

Figure 1.6
An orthopantomogram (OPG) showing the mixed dentition of deciduous (d) and permanent (p) teeth in a 10-year-old female twin.

Table 1.1

Timing of primary teeth emergence in Australian twins (months)[1]

	Right				Left			
	n	mean	SD	CV	n	mean	SD	CV
	Maxillary							
central incisor	207	10.8	2.0	18.8	206	10.8	2.2	20.4
lateral incisor	199	12.3	2.9	23.4	201	12.1	2.9	24.1
canine	136	19.3	3.5	18.3	139	19.3	3.5	18.1
first molar	179	15.9	2.4	15.0	180	15.9	2.4	15.1
second molar	69	27.9	4.4	15.8	70	27.7	4.4	16.1
	Mandibular							
central incisor	204	8.6	2.0	23.7	206	8.7	2.1	24.8
lateral incisor	189	14.2	3.3	23.1	185	13.9	3.4	24.1
canine	135	19.9	3.7	18.6	138	19.7	3.9	20.0
first molar	175	16.7	2.5	15.0	175	16.5	2.4	14.4
second molar	73	27.1	3.8	14.1	72	26.7	3.7	13.8

[1] Woodroffe et al., 2010. Data for boys and girls combined. SD = standard deviation; CV = coefficient of variation (CV = 100(SD/mean)).

until the late teens. The third molars are prone to impaction due to lack of space in the jaws. There is considerable variation in the timing of emergence of teeth between individuals. For example, maxillary (upper) central incisors may emerge between 5.8 and 9.1 years in boys with a median value of 7.4 years (Table 1.2).

The permanent teeth tend to emerge a little earlier in girls than boys, with the biggest difference being for the canines (Table 1.3).

Fortunately for some people, their third molars do not form at all, so they are not faced with having to decide whether their 'wisdom teeth' should be extracted. The biological reason for congenitally missing teeth, also referred to as hypodontia or dental agenesis, is one question that we have addressed in our studies but there is still much more to learn.

Table 1.2

Median emergence times (years) for permanent teeth in Australian males, including 5th and 95th percentiles[1]

Tooth			Median	5th percentile	95th percentile
Males					
Maxillary		1	7.43	5.79	9.06
		2	8.61	6.36	10.86
		3	11.81	9.46	14.15
		4	11.28	8.94	13.62
		5	12.05	9.67	14.43
		6	6.71	5.05	8.37
		7	12.68	10.28	15.08
Mandibular		1	6.63	4.96	8.29
		2	7.77	5.97	9.58
		3	11.02	8.94	13.10
		4	11.15	9.01	13.29
		5	12.11	9.68	14.54
		6	6.63	4.96	8.30
		7	12.15	9.83	14.48

[1]Diamanti and Townsend, 2003. Median is the 50th percentile: 5% of children fall below the 5th percentile and 5% above the 95th percentile.

Table 1.3

Median emergence times (years), for permanent teeth in Australian females, including 5th and 95th percentiles

Tooth		Median	5th percentile	95th percentile
Females				
Maxillary	1	7.17	5.64	8.69
	2	8.24	5.99	10.49
	3	11.23	8.80	13.65
	4	10.77	8.58	12.96
	5	11.67	9.17	14.17
	6	6.57	4.84	8.30
	7	12.30	9.90	14.70
Mandibular	1	6.38	4.77	7.99
	2	7.47	5.67	9.28
	3	10.11	8.03	12.20
	4	10.59	8.45	12.73
	5	11.66	9.11	14.22
	6	6.42	4.86	7.98
	7	11.75	9.42	14.07

[1]Diamanti and Townsend, 2003. Median is the 50th percentile: 5% of children fall below the 5th percentile and 5% above the 95th percentile.

WHAT ARE THE MAIN FEATURES OF THE PRIMARY AND PERMANENT TEETH?

There are usually twenty primary or deciduous teeth in the human dentition, comprising a central incisor, lateral incisor, canine and two molars in each quadrant (quarter) of the mouth. The primary teeth tend to be smaller than their permanent successors, with slightly different crown shapes. Their roots are more slender and flared in the molar region, and they undergo a process of resorption that leads to the teeth being exfoliated just prior to the emergence of their permanent successor. A full permanent dentition comprises thirty-two teeth, with central and lateral incisors, canine, two premolars and three molars in each quadrant. The incisor crowns display relatively flat incisal edges, whereas the canine has a single cusp. The premolars often have two cusps on their occlusal surfaces, while molar teeth tend to be four- or five-cusped (Figure 1.7).

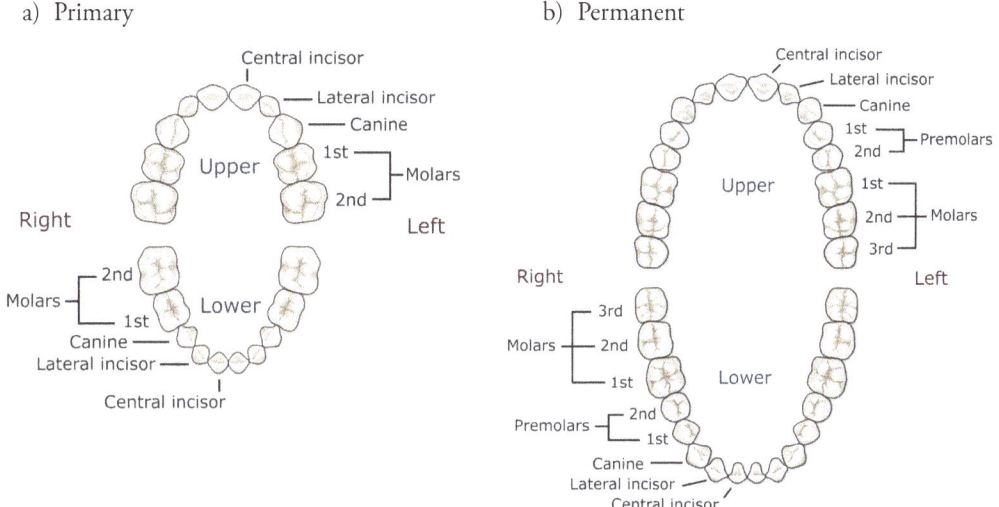

Figure 1.7
Diagrams showing (a) primary and (b) permanent human dentitions.

As mentioned, sometimes teeth may fail to develop, leading to a reduced number of teeth in the arch and often spacing between those teeth that are present in the mouth. As shown in Figure 1.8, if one member of a pair of monozygotic twins has a missing tooth or teeth, the other member is also likely to be affected. However, the expression of missing teeth often differs between the two, suggesting that epigenetic and/or environmental factors are involved.

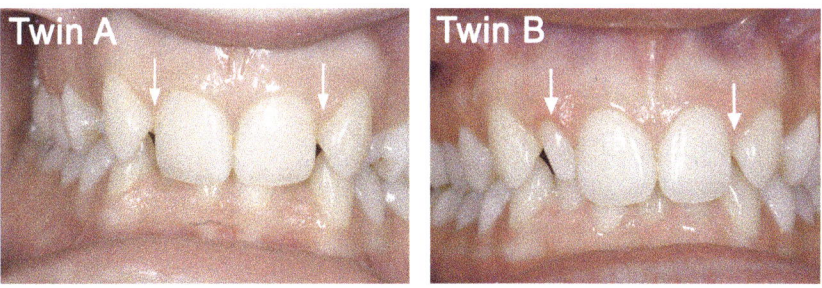

Figure 1.8
Monozygotic female twins where Twin A (left) displays bilateral agenesis of the maxillary lateral incisors (both upper lateral incisors have failed to form); and Twin B (right) has a peg-shaped maxillary right lateral incisor and agenesis of the maxillary left lateral incisor.

Occasionally, there may be an extra tooth or teeth present in the mouth — these are referred to as supernumerary teeth. These teeth may emerge into the mouth or remain within the jaws. If they are associated with pathology they may be extracted. Again, if one member of a monozygotic twin pair has a supernumerary tooth, the other is also likely to have one, but the expression often differs between the twins. In the case shown in Figure 1.9, one twin has one supernumerary and the other has two.

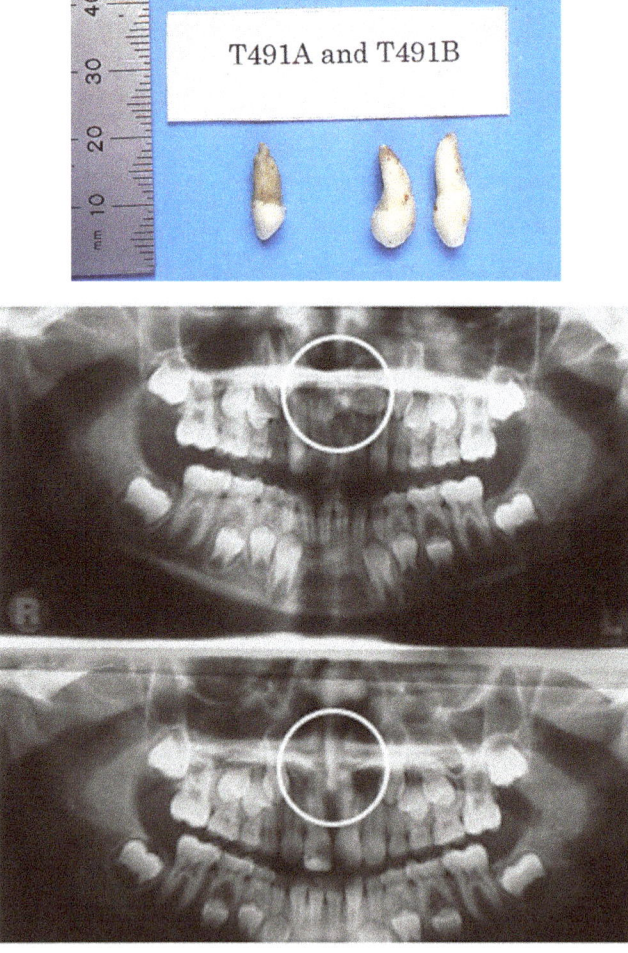

Figure 1.9
Supernumerary teeth of a pair of monozygotic twin boys and panoramic radiographs showing the location of the teeth prior to extraction (circled).

A tour of the mouth

How are the teeth arranged in the oral cavity?

The teeth are arranged in dental arches that are often parabolic in shape but they may vary from a very broad ovoid shape to a narrow U-shaped arrangement. The upper and lower teeth normally fit together to facilitate the functions of the biting, chewing and speaking. We are all aware that sometimes the arrangement of the teeth varies from what is considered normal — for example, a buck-toothed arrangement where the upper anterior teeth protrude anteriorly in front of the lowers. At the other extreme, there can be instances where the lower dental arch protrudes in front of the upper, producing a so-called crossbite arrangement of the teeth. These extreme variations in the relationships between upper and lower teeth can have significant effects on appearance (aesthetics), as well as function, and they are commonly referred to as malocclusions.

Most individuals display some variation from a so-called ideal dental occlusion, so we prefer to use the term 'occlusal variation' to encompass everyone, rather than focusing on so-called malocclusions and comparing them to 'normal' occlusions. Interestingly, we have found that variation in some occlusal features, such as anterior overbite and overjet, is not influenced by genetic factors as much as variation in others — for example, arch dimensions. Figure 1.10 (overleaf) shows good alignment of teeth in a pair of monozygotic twins and crowded teeth in another pair of monozygotic twins.

Tooth notation

There are several notations that have been developed to assist dentists who are charting the teeth that are present in their patients' mouths. One is the Fédération Dentaire Internationale (FDI) notation and another is Palmer's notation. These notations are often used in tables and figures in research papers when referring to teeth and so we provide a brief summary of each here.

The FDI notation uses a two-digit system and can be adapted easily to computer charts. The first digit refers to the quadrant in the mouth in which the tooth is located. For the permanent dentition, the quadrants are numbered from 1 to 4 commencing with the upper right quadrant, which is denoted quadrant 1. The numbering then continues in a clockwise direction (from the dentist's viewpoint of the patient's mouth)

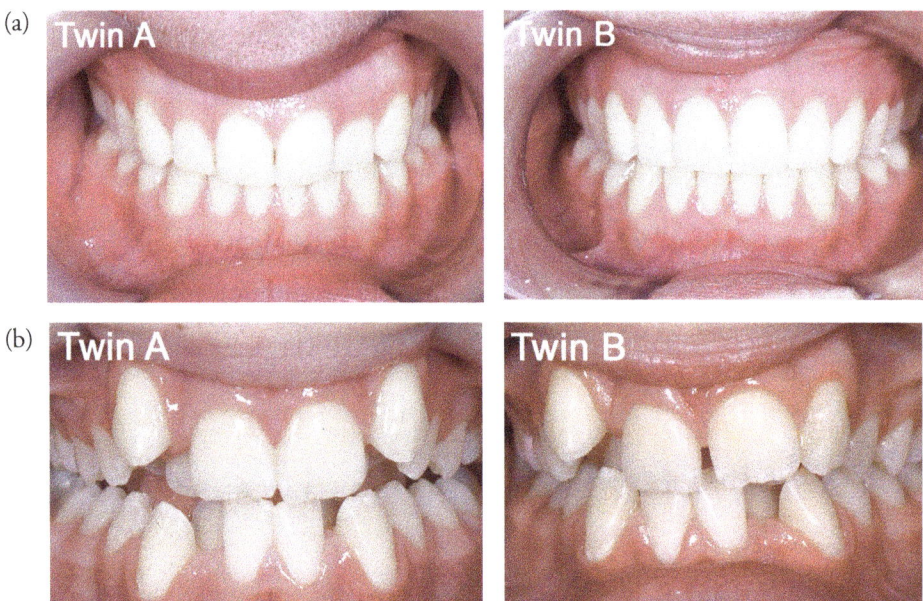

Figure 1.10
(a) A pair of monozygotic twins showing good occlusion and (b) a pair of monozygotic twins showing crowding.

to the upper left (quadrant 2), then the lower left (quadrant 3), then the lower right (quadrant 4). Continuing on for the primary or deciduous dentition, the upper right quadrant is labelled 5, the upper left is 6, the lower left is 7 and the lower right is 8. The second digit identifies the tooth within the quadrant. The permanent teeth are numbered from 1 to 8 in each quadrant and the primary teeth are numbered from 1 to 5. The numbering commences in the front of the mouth and proceeds posteriorly toward the molars. The numbers are pronounced separately, so that a permanent upper left first molar tooth would be labelled as a 26, pronounced 'two six' (Figure 1.11).

Palmer's notation also divides the mouth into quadrants or quarters, but it employs a diagrammatic representation of the four quadrants using a cross. The permanent teeth are numbered from 1 to 8 in each quadrant, beginning in the midline, whereas the primary teeth are identified by the letters, A to E (Figure 1.12). Individual teeth are denoted by either a number (for the permanent dentition) or by a letter (for the primary dentition), which is enclosed in the two sides of the cross that indicate the quadrant (as shown in Figure 1.12).

A tour of the mouth

a) Primary

b) Permanent

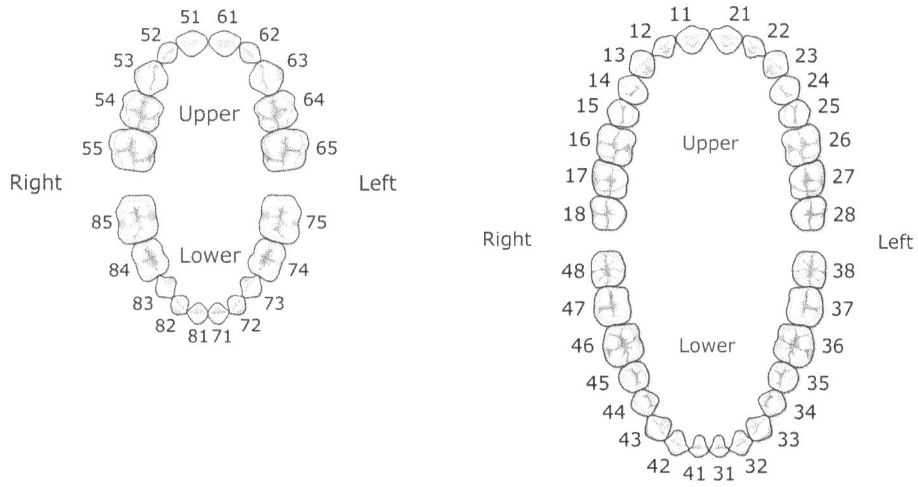

Figure 1.11
The Fédération Dentaire Internationale (FDI) notation for charting the (a) primary and (b) permanent dentitions.

a) Primary

b) Permanent

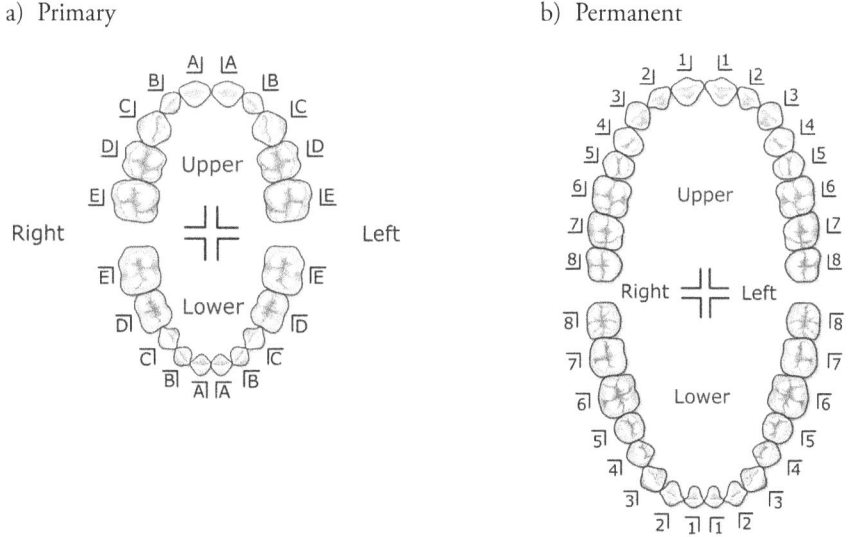

Figure 1.12
Palmer's notation for (a) primary and (b) permanent dentitions.

What are the main tissues that make up a tooth?

The crowns of teeth are covered with a highly mineralised, hard and brittle substance referred to as enamel. This tissue is composed of hydroxyapatite crystals that are arranged in rods to form a 'grain' structure, which means that enamel tends to fracture along the line of the rods. Because of its high inorganic content, enamel is particularly susceptible to dissolution by acids, whether these are produced by bacteria in dental plaque around the teeth or by ingested foods and drinks that are acidic. The thickness of the enamel varies in different parts of the crown, being thickest in the regions of the cusps and the incisal edges and thinnest in the cervical regions.

Dentine forms most of the tooth and it is a tubular, mineralised tissue that is not as hard as enamel. In contrast to enamel, dentine contains the processes of living cells, referred to as odontoblasts, so it is a vital tissue that can elicit a painful response if exposed to the oral cavity, or in response to the spread of dental decay (also referred to as dental caries). The dentine and the enamel of teeth contact at the dentino-enamel junction (DEJ), which represents the original site where the inner part of the enamel organ (the inner enamel epithelium) and the dental papilla were next to one another during dental development.

The inner part of teeth is filled with a soft connective tissue referred to as the dental pulp. This tissue comprises cells, fibres, blood vessels, nerves and ground substance. If the pulp of a vital tooth is exposed, either through trauma or during restorative treatment, a small amount of blood will be visible. Teeth with exposed pulps are usually highly sensitive (Figure 1.13).

A thin layer of cement covers the roots of teeth, and the roots are attached to the surrounding bone of the jaws (alveolar bone) by a system of fibres referred to as the periodontal membrane or ligament. This structure normally enables a small amount of mobility of each tooth in its socket but, if the membrane is broken down due to inflammatory processes (periodontitis) and there is also resorption of alveolar bone, then the tooth can become more mobile.

On radiographs of teeth, the pulp tissue appears dark (radiolucent) compared with the lighter appearance of the calcified dentine and enamel (radiopaque). Figure 1.14 shows teeth in varying stages of development, with two restored with radiopaque fillings.

A tour of the mouth

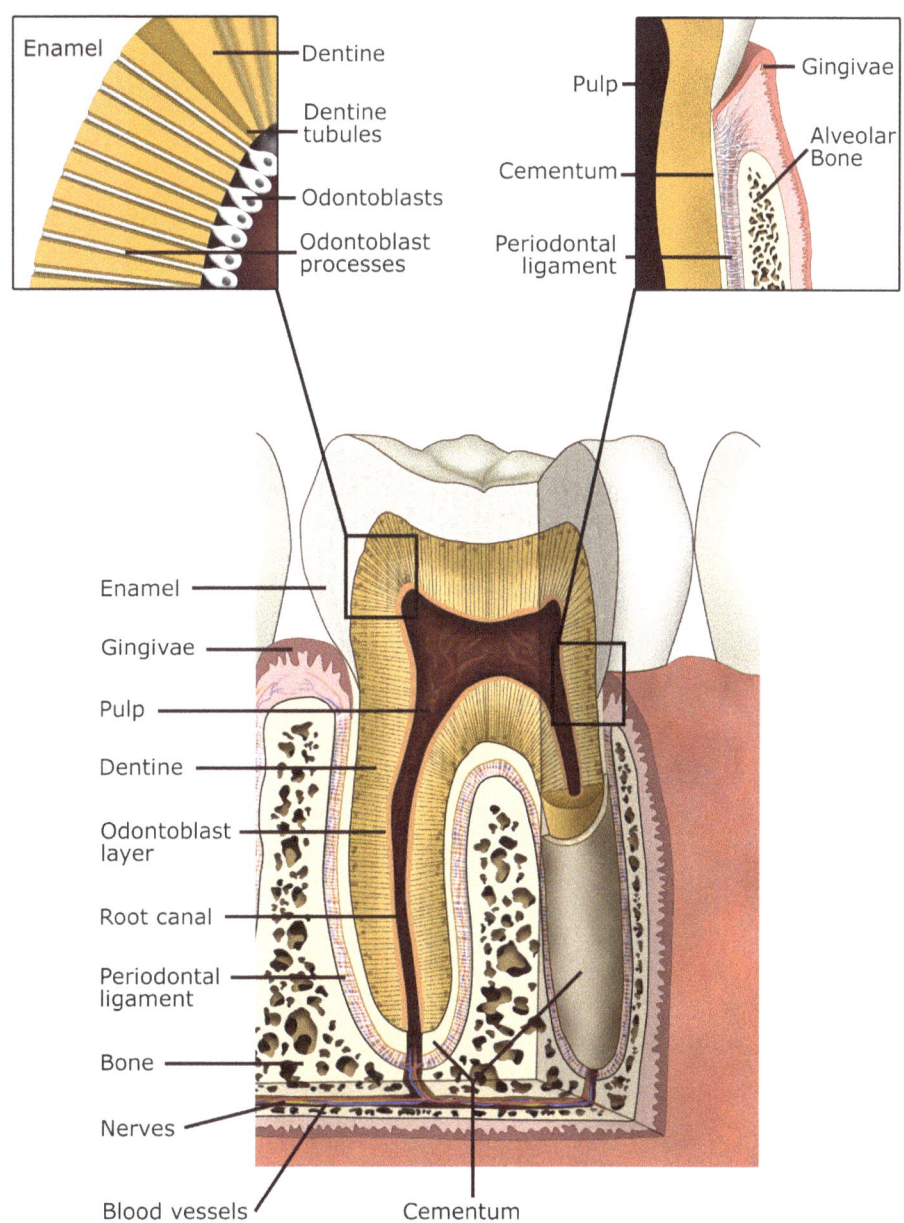

Figure 1.13
The main tissues that make up and support a tooth.

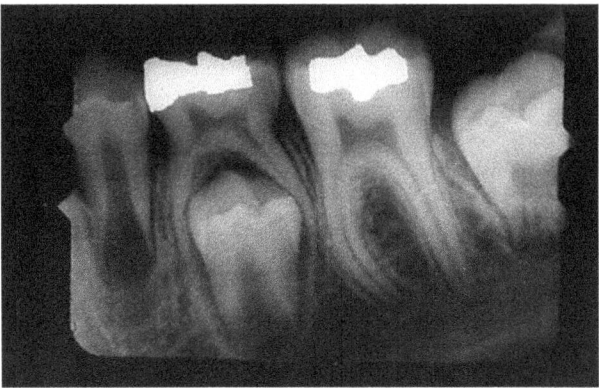

Figure 1.14
A bite wing radiograph showing the developing dentition. The occlusal surfaces of the molars have been restored and the fillings appear as bright white areas. A developing permanent premolar can be seen under a primary molar.

The overall size of dental crowns is determined by a combination of the thickness of the enamel and dentine, and the size of the underlying pulp chamber. These structures can be visualised on radiographs and, provided these images are standardised, measurements can be made from them. A question that continues to evoke interest is the extent to which each of these tissues contributes to the final size and shape of dental crowns. For example, we know that the dental crowns of males tend to be larger, on average, than those of females — but why? Recent applications of three-dimensional (3D) imaging techniques — for example, 3D CT scanning — are now helping to unravel these questions. 3D imaging also enables researchers to explore the inner aspects of teeth, to see to what extent the external appearance of a particular tooth is a reflection of the blueprint laid down during development at the site of the future junction between the enamel and the dentine, the dentino-enamel junction (DEJ).

How can we study dental morphology?

Traditionally, the size and shape of teeth have been recorded using hand-held callipers to measure certain dimensions on dental models — for example, the maximum mesiodistal and buccolingual crown diameters (Figure 1.15) — or by describing certain features according to their degree of expression, such as grooves, pits, small cusps or large cusps. While these methods have yielded considerable information about the nature and extent of variation in the dentition within and between populations, they are relatively crude measures that fail to capture much of the variability in tooth surfaces. More recently, high-precision two-dimensional (2D) and 3D imaging systems have been applied to record not only traditional measurements but also to define new dental phenotypes, including intercuspal distances (Figure 1.15), crown contours, areas and volumes.

We have coined the term 'dental phenomics' to refer to this new era of studying dental phenotypes both intensively and extensively (Townsend et al., 2012; Yong et al., 2014). It is our belief that these sophisticated measuring systems will prove to be valuable in building up large sets of data that will define both the external and internal morphologies of teeth. If these new dental phenotypes can be recorded in large samples of twins, and we can then apply modern methods of genome-wide scanning, it should be possible to locate and identify the key genes involved in human dental development. Such discoveries will have major implications for many fields of

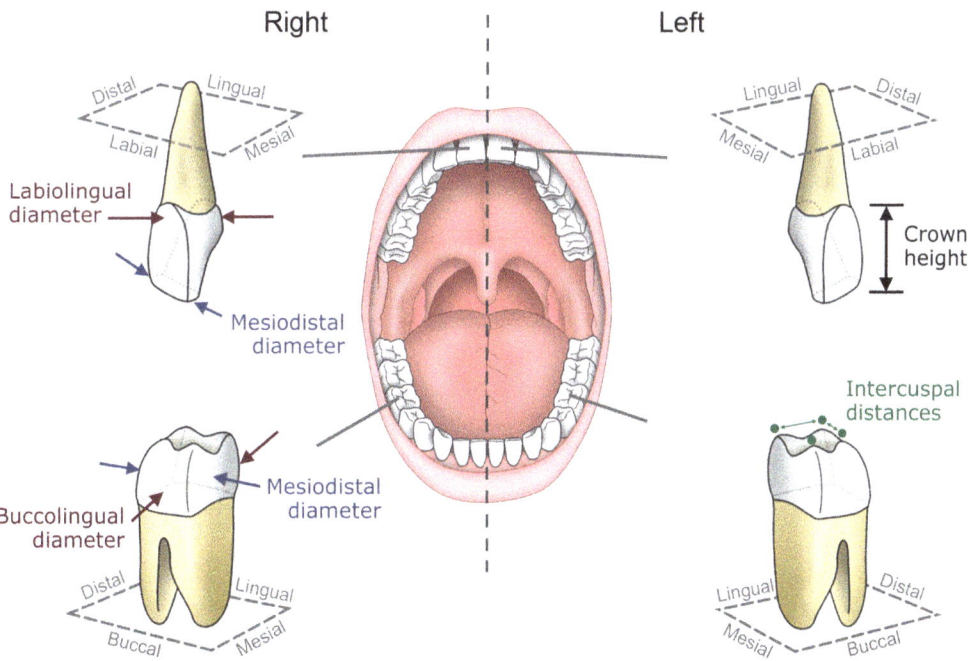

Figure 1.15
Diagrammatic representation of tooth surfaces and some selected measurements.

research and also, ultimately, for practising dentists faced with treating individuals presenting with various oral diseases and disorders.

WHY IS THE DENTITION SUCH A GOOD MODEL SYSTEM FOR STUDYING DEVELOPMENT?

The dentition provides a unique model system for studying developmental events occurring over an extended period of time, from early on prenatally through until adolescence. As we have seen, development of the primary incisors commences in the first few weeks of life, followed by the other primary teeth and then the permanent teeth. Each tooth passes through a series of well-defined developmental stages, beginning with rapid growth of soft tissue, then subsequent crown and root calcification. Final crown morphology is determined well before each tooth emerges into the oral cavity and does not change thereafter, apart from the effects of tooth wear and restorative procedures. Therefore, by studying final crown size and shape, and applying knowledge of the timing and sequence of dental development, one can attempt to retrospectively elucidate the nature of tissue interactions and disturbances in early growth which may have affected final crown morphology.

The stability and durability of dental crowns are particularly valuable features in genetic studies because they allow comparisons of tooth size and shape to be made between related and non-related individuals irrespective of their age. Investigations of the associations between teeth in the primary and permanent dentitions of individuals help to clarify co-ordinating mechanisms that may be operating and to disclose possible pleiotropic effects of genes — that is, genes that appear to affect more than one feature. Comparisons can also be made between upper and lower teeth, between teeth within a particular tooth class — for example, the molar series — as well as between corresponding teeth on right and left sides, so-called antimeric teeth.

Apart from obtaining dental impressions from many of the twins enrolled in our studies to enable stone models (or casts) to be constructed, we have also obtained fingerprints and palm-prints. The reason for doing this has been that both teeth and fingerprints form as a result of interactions between a surface epithelial layer and underlying mesenchymal tissue. Furthermore, once fingerprints are formed, they do not change in their appearance, similar to teeth. Also, it is possible to compare the different patterns of expression of the fingerprints between different fingers of one hand or between right and left hands. Although we have collected extensive dermatoglyphic records from twins and their families, we have only just begun to analyse them to see whether there are common co-ordinating mechanisms and possibly common genes involved in establishing the patterns we observe in both teeth and fingerprints.

What are some of the common developmental anomalies affecting teeth?

There are many anomalies that can affect the teeth, including variations in number, size and shape. As mentioned previously, certain teeth may fail to form in some individuals. Most commonly the third molars are affected, but other teeth that may display agenesis or hypodontia are the permanent upper lateral incisors and the second premolars. Figure 1.16 shows panoramic radiographs of a pair of monozygotic twins who both show evidence of missing teeth, but the expression varies between the two. For example, Twin A has a missing lower right second premolar (arrowed) whereas this tooth is present in Twin B. It appears that both twins have developing lower third molars but missing upper third molars (circles). These differences in expression of missing teeth between the members of a monozygotic twin pair provide further support for the role of epigenetic and/or environmental influences on dental development.

In contrast to missing teeth, occasionally there may be extra, or so-called supernumerary, teeth present (Figure 1.17). Commonly these occur behind the upper central incisors, referred to as a mesiodens, but there may also be supernumerary premolars or molars. Interestingly, missing teeth are more common in females than males, whereas supernumeraries are more common in males. There is a link between tooth size and shape, and the presence or absence of teeth, and this has been described elegantly by Alan Brook and colleagues (2014). Alan is currently an Adjunct Professor in the School of Dentistry at the University of Adelaide and a valued and active member of our research group.

Variations in size of teeth include very small teeth, so-called microdontia, and very large teeth, referred to as macrodontia (Figure 1.18). These anomalies may involve a single tooth within the dentition, or many or all teeth may be affected. A commonly described example of a small tooth is the microdont upper lateral incisor, which is also associated with other variations of this tooth, including peg-shaped upper lateral incisors and agenesis of upper laterals (Figure 1.18).

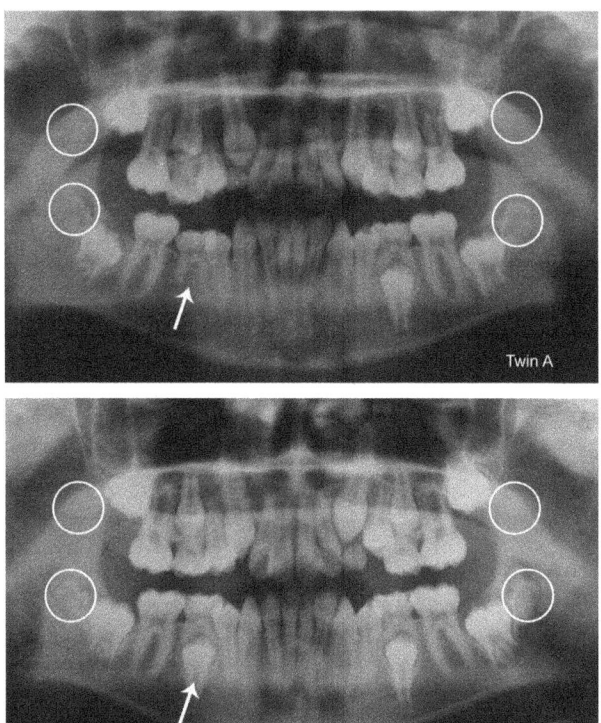

Figure 1.16
Panoramic radiographs of a pair of monozygotic twins showing missing teeth. The circled areas indicate the regions where third molars would normally develop. The arrows point to regions where permanent second premolars usually form. Reproduced with permission from the Australian Dental Journal (Hughes et al., 2014).

Other dental features that have been described extensively by dental anthropologists include the following: Carabelli trait, which varies in expression from pits and grooves of various types to cusps of different sizes on the mesio-lingual surface of primary upper second molars and permanent upper first molars mainly; small cusps or tubercles on the lingual aspect of anterior teeth; shovelling of incisor teeth with marked expression of the marginal ridges; and extra cusps on molar teeth, such as accessory cusp 7 which appears between the lingual cusps of lower molars (Figure 1.19). Standard plaques have been constructed to enable researchers to reliably score the different expressions of these features on dental models. It is then possible to

A tour of the mouth

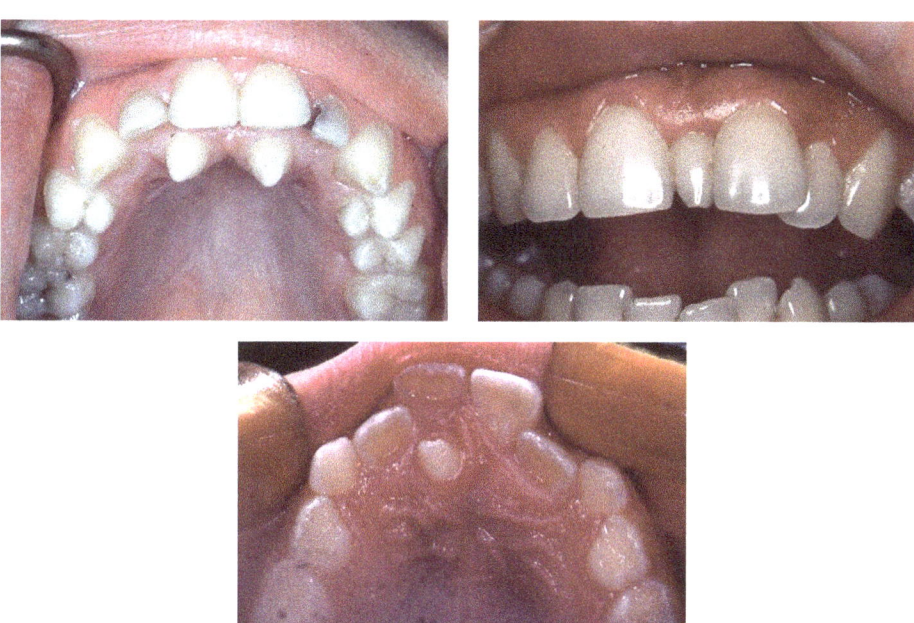

Figure 1.17
Examples of supernumerary teeth in the upper incisor region.

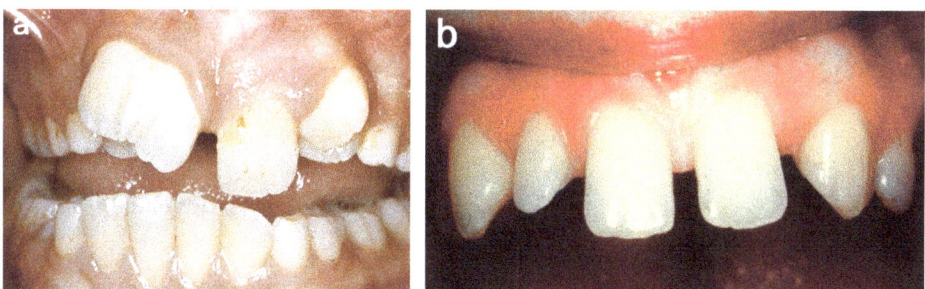

Figure 1.18
(a) A patient with a supernumerary upper left lateral incisor, a megadont/double upper right central incisor and generalised large tooth size, and (b) a patient with hypodontia of the upper left lateral incisor and microdontia of the upper right lateral incisor. The upper central incisors also show a reduction in shape from the average. Reproduced with permission from the Australian Dental Journal (Brook et al., 2014).

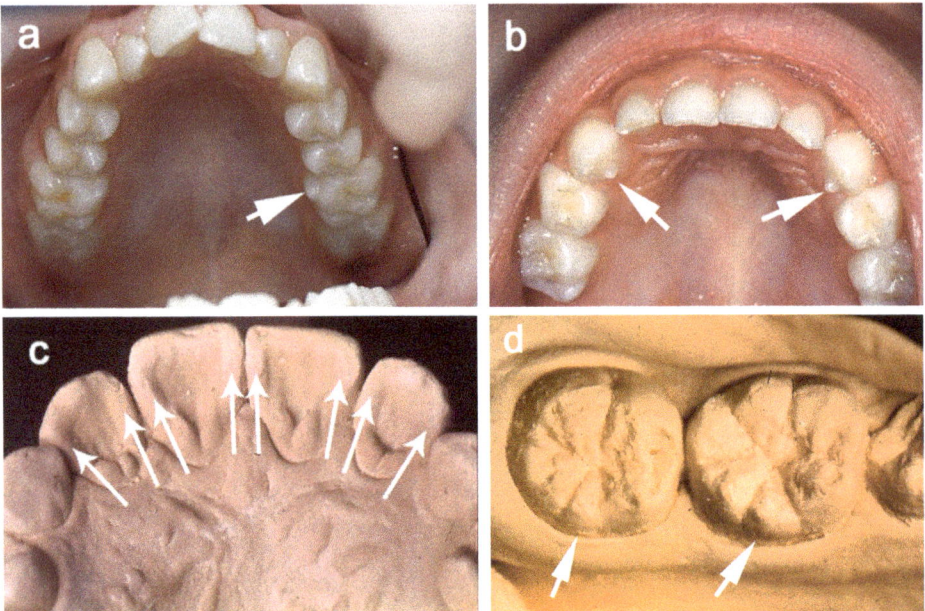

Figure 1.19
Dental features including (a) Carabelli trait, (b) lingual tubercles, (c) shovel-shaped incisors and (d) extra cusps on molar teeth.

compare their appearance in related individuals to try to unravel the contributions of genetic and environmental influences to observed variation.

Anomalies of tooth structure may affect any of the dental tissues. For example, developmental disturbances may lead to poorly formed enamel (enamel hypoplasia), which presents clinically as white patches, pits or grooves on dental crowns (Figure 1.20). Hypoplasia may be due to a mutation of one of the genes involved in the formation of enamel (amelogenesis) or it may result from an environmental disturbance during dental development, such as a viral illness or fever. The distribution of structural anomalies across the dentition, together with a patient's history, gives the clinician some insight into the possible causes. For instance, enamel hypoplastic defects that affect all teeth in both dentitions are likely to have a genetic cause (aetiology), whereas a single affected tooth suggests some local environmental disturbance. Some types of enamel hypoplasia that present as linear defects on the tooth crown or pitting can be studied on dental models, provided the models are of good quality.

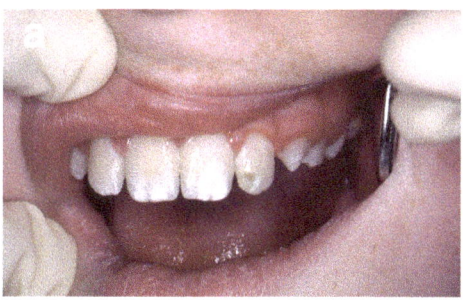 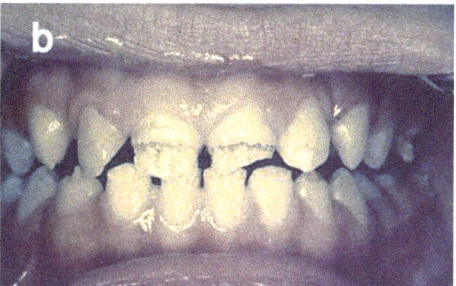

Figure 1.20
Two examples of enamel hypoplasia, presenting as (a) white patches on the central incisors and a localised defect on the upper left lateral incisor and (b) generalised pitting and grooving.

WHAT ARE THE MOST IMPORTANT DISEASES OR PROBLEMS THAT CAN AFFECT OUR TEETH?

The most common dental diseases, which affect most of us to some extent, are dental decay (caries) and gum disease (gingivitis). Dental caries refers to the progressive localised demineralisation and destruction of tooth tissues (the word 'caries' is derived from Latin and means 'rottenness'). Dental caries results from a prolonged imbalance of factors that favour demineralisation over those that favour mineralisation. The factors that need to be considered include the 'host', particularly their saliva and the structure and morphology of their teeth; the oral microflora, particularly the composition of the dental plaque that adheres to the teeth; and the diet, which forms the substrate for the bacteria in dental plaque.

Bacteria in dental plaque and refined carbohydrates in the diet interact with protective factors, including saliva and good oral hygiene, to determine the balance between demineralisation and remineralisation. Repeated pH drops (due to acid production by plaque bacteria) can lead to demineralisation of enamel, with the frequency of these drops in pH being very important (Figure 1.21).

Inflammation of the gums around the teeth is referred to as gingivitis. Clear signs of gingivitis are evidence of blood on a toothbrush after cleaning, or bleeding from around the necks of the teeth when an oral health professional gently probes the gingival crevice around the neck of a tooth. More severe inflammation leads to

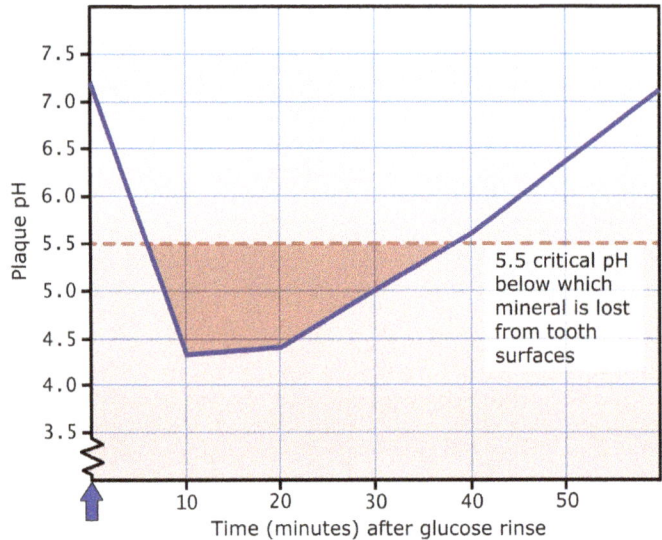

Figure 1.21
This graph, referred to as a Stephan curve, shows the drop in pH that occurs in dental plaque after rinsing the mouth with a sugar solution. Below the critical pH, enamel will demineralise.

red, puffy, swollen gums. In a fairly small percentage of individuals, the process of inflammation may extend to involve the supporting tissues of the tooth (periodontal ligament or membrane), causing loss of attachment of the gingival tissues to the tooth, apical migration of the epithelial attachment, pocket formation, gingival recession, loss of alveolar bone, mobility of teeth and possible loss of teeth.

As with dental caries, periodontitis has a complex aetiology. Basically, bacteria in plaque around the necks of teeth produce toxic products which may cause inflammation of the periodontal tissues. However, the balance between bacteria and the body's defence system is very important. That is, bacteria are essential agents, but their presence is in itself insufficient. Host factors must be involved if the disease is to develop and progress. Figure 1.22 shows the teeth and gums of a pair of monozygotic twins who both show evidence of gum disease (gingivitis) and dental decay (dental caries).

While genetic factors are clearly involved in both of these diseases, their aetiologies are complex. The application of different twin models offers many advantages in exploring the relative contributions of genetic, epigenetic and environmental contributions to observed variation in these common dental diseases.

A tour of the mouth

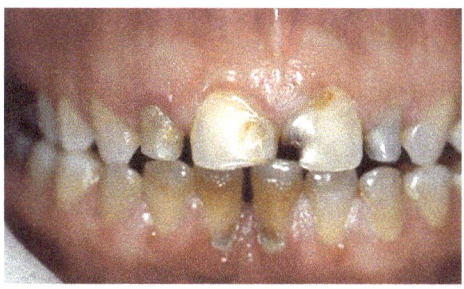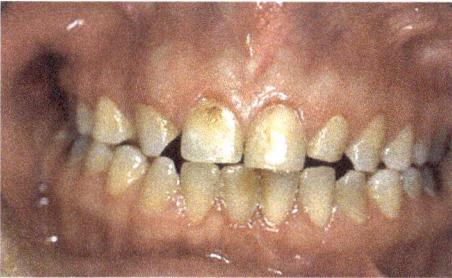

Figure 1.22
Intra-oral photographs of a pair of monozygotic twins, aged 38 years, showing evidence of inflammation of the gums (gingivitis) and also dental decay (dental caries), with associated build-up of dental plaque around the teeth.

IS THERE A RELATIONSHIP BETWEEN ORAL HEALTH AND GENERAL HEALTH?

There has been an increasing realisation over the past decade or so that oral health and general health are intimately related. We know that many systemic diseases have oral manifestations, with oral signs and symptoms often being the first indicators of disease. The oral cavity is also an entry point for various microbial infections that can affect general health. Not only is the mouth a potential site of entry for micro-organisms, it may also harbour microbial infections — for example, dental caries and periodontal diseases — which have the potential to affect general health.

Associations have now been documented between periodontal diseases and several chronic systemic diseases or problems, including cardiovascular disease, diabetes and respiratory disease, highlighting the fact that oral diseases are not merely localised problems but can have significant implications for our general health and well-being (Figure 1.23).

Clearly, future discoveries about genetic, epigenetic and environmental contributions to oral health and disease will have much wider ramifications than many researchers and clinicians may have thought in the past. So, while our earlier studies of twins and their families were focused on dental development and morphology, our more recent investigations have broadened to consider the way in which the microbiome of the oral cavity — that is, all of the bacteria living in the mouth — is established and how this is associated with an individual's susceptibility to future disease.

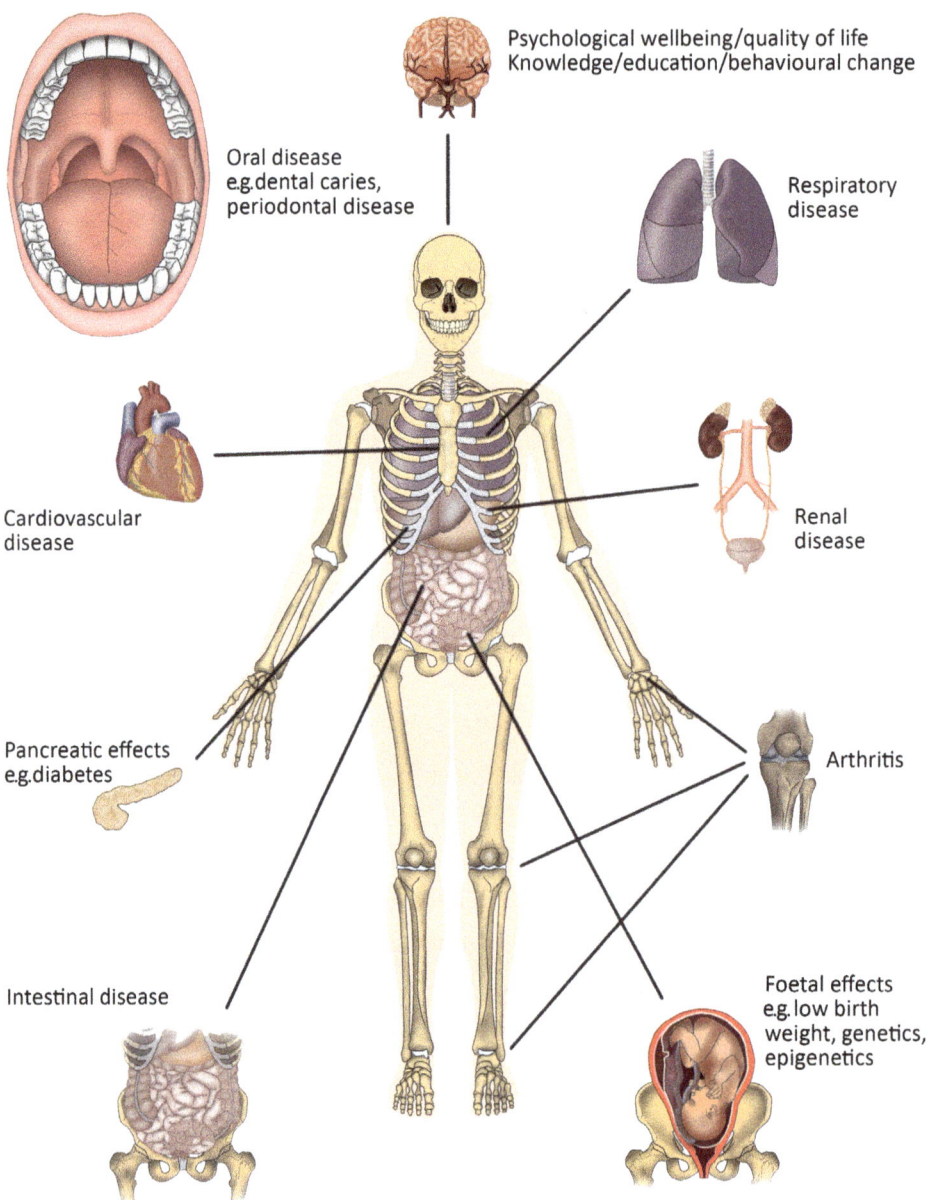

Figure 1.23
Diagrammatic representation of reported associations between oral disease and systemic diseases and disorders.

Interestingly, a recent investigation of the placental microbiome in 320 subjects showed that the placental profiles were most similar to the human oral microbiome (Aagaard et al., 2014). These findings are particularly significant given the known association between periodontal disease and increased risk of pre-term birth and low birthweight.

WHY MIGHT TWINS' TEETH LOOK THE SAME OR DIFFERENT?

Parents of twins are often curious to know whether their twins' teeth will look the same or not. Given that there seems to be a relatively strong genetic contribution to variation in the size, shape, arrangement and development of teeth (which we will discuss further in subsequent chapters), one would expect that monozygotic twins (also called identical twins) should display similar dental features. Indeed, this is generally what is found. Sometimes, the teeth of a pair of monozygotic twins cannot be distinguished from one another, even after very close inspection or measurement. In fact, we have come across examples where the upper dental arch of one co-twin can be matched (or occluded) precisely with the lower arch of the other co-twin. This is quite remarkable given the number of interacting factors that are involved both in producing the upper and lower dental arches and in designing them so that they occlude together perfectly.

However, we have noted many examples where the teeth of monozygotic co-twins can differ in appearance, sometimes quite markedly. For example, there may be differences in the size and shape of one or more teeth, in the shapes of the dental arches, or differences in the number or position of extra or missing teeth. These differences may be due to 'environmental' factors which act differentially on the members of the twin pair. Alternatively, they may be due to differences in the way in which the genes of the monozygotic co-twins are expressed — referred to as epigenetic factors. A specific example of differences between monozygotic co-twins, referred to as mirror imaging, occurs when one twin 'mirrors' the other for one or more dental features. In these cases, the right side of one twin will match the left side of the other and vice-versa (Figures 1.24 and 1.25). We will give further examples of monozygotic co-twins with very similar and dissimilar teeth, including some fascinating examples of mirror imaging, in the following chapters.

If twins are dizygotic (also called fraternal twins) they will only share 50 per cent of their genes on average. These twins are no more closely related than siblings

Twin Studies

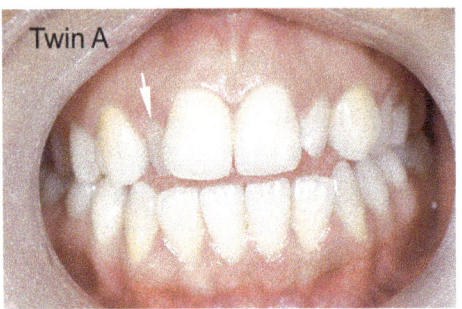
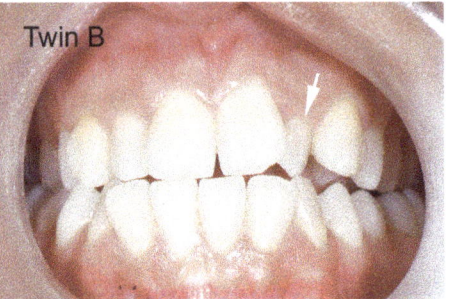

Figure 1.24
A pair of monozygotic twins showing mirror imaging in the crowding of their anterior teeth. Twin A's upper right central incisor has crossed over the upper right lateral and Twin B's upper left central incisor has partially obscured the upper left lateral.

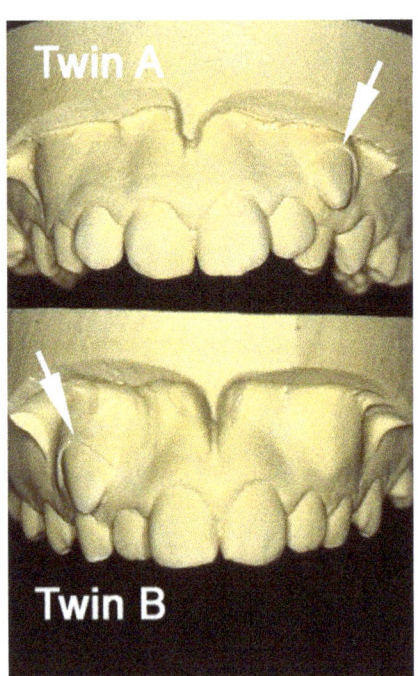

Figure 1.25
Dental models of a pair of monozygotic twins with mirror-imaged emergence of the upper canine.

A tour of the mouth

and, therefore, they may share some common dental features, in terms of size, shape, arrangement, and timing of development, but they will usually be fairly easy to distinguish (Figure 1.26).

A pair of dizygotic twins may share more than 50 per cent of their genes and, when this occurs, they may have very similar dental features. It is well established that males have, on average, larger teeth than females, although the magnitude of the differences is only a few tenths of a millimetre. This feature is referred to as sexual dimorphism. This means that we would expect the teeth of males from dizygotic opposite-sex pairs (boy-girl twin pairs) to be larger on average than those of their female co-twins (Figure 1.27).

While this seems to be true, we have found that the extent of sexual dimorphism in these twin pairs is less than expected, due to an increase in the size of the females' teeth. The most likely reason for this effect is that the females are affected in utero by male hormones produced by the male co-twin. This effect is explained by the 'Twin Testosterone Transfer (TTT) hypothesis', and our studies of tooth size in twins

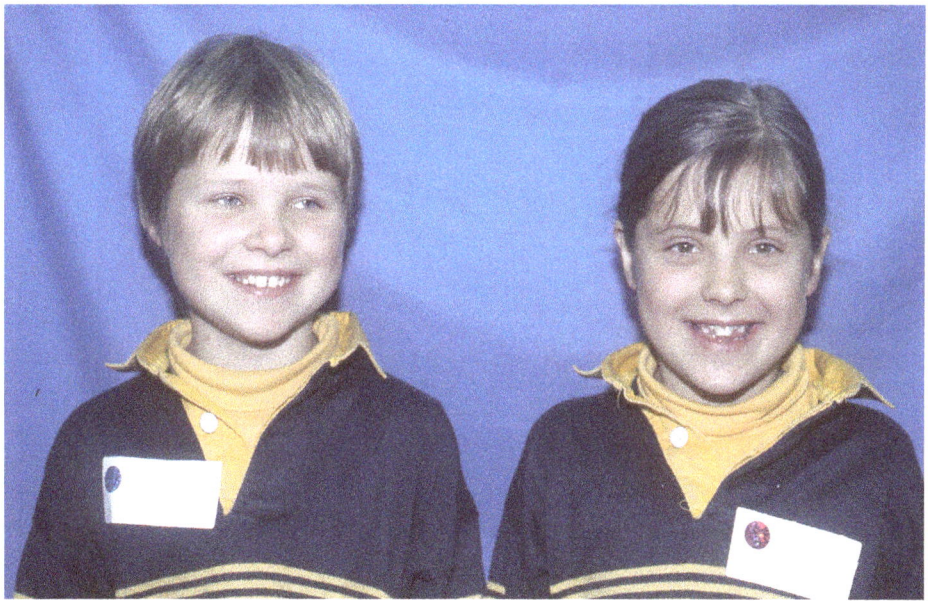

Figure 1.26
A pair of dizygotic (fraternal) twin girls with different hair, eye colour, facial features and stages of dental development.

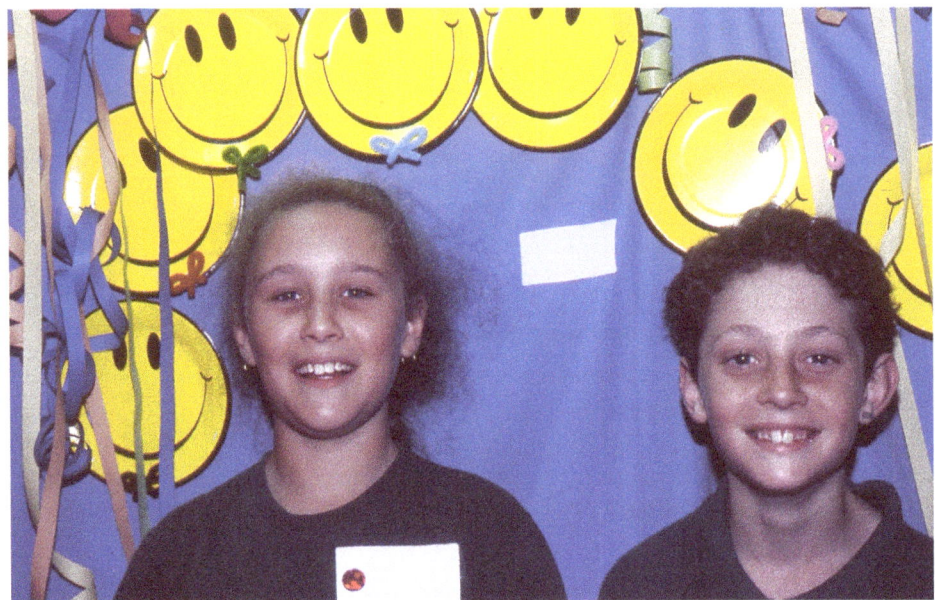

Figure 1.27
A pair of opposite-sex dizygotic twins.

provide one of the strongest pieces of evidence in support of the TTT hypothesis based on a physical feature. We will discuss this finding further in Chapter Five.

We hope that you have found this first chapter informative, in providing some basic dental terminology and brief descriptions about dental development, as well as common oral diseases and abnormalities. Dental research involving twins is a relatively recent innovation, whereas reports of twinning and the effects of twins on those around them have existed since humans first recorded their history. To provide some context for a more detailed description of our studies of Australian twins, Chapter Two provides an historical perspective of twin studies in general and with particular reference to how twins were seen by those involved in twin exploration. Some of the key studies that have been carried out in the past on the teeth and faces of twins are described in Chapter Three. Chapters Four to Six then provide details about our own studies of Australian twins and their families, based in the School of Dentistry at the University of Adelaide. We have studied three main cohorts of twins over the past thirty years, referred to as Cohort 1, Cohort 2 and Cohort 3, and the main investigations and findings related to each of these groups are provided in Chapters Four, Five and Six respectively. Also in Chapter Six, we look to the future and consider where our studies of twins are going. Chapter Seven provides a full listing of publications and theses arising from our twin studies, followed by a section containing a glossary of terms. There is also an Appendix that includes a list of colleagues, visiting researchers, collaborators and key contributors, as well as a gallery of photographs of some of the researchers, twins and their families.

References

Aagaard K, Ma J, Antony KM, Ganu R, Petrosino J, Versalovic J (2014). The placenta harbors a unique microbiome. *Sci Transl Med* 6:237ra65.

Brook AH, Jernvall J, Smith RN, Hughes TE, Townsend GC (2014). The dentition: the outcomes of morphogenesis leading to variations of tooth number, size and shape. *Aust Dent J* 59 (1 Suppl):131-142.

Diamanti J, Townsend GC (2003). New standards for permanent tooth emergence in Australian children. *Aust Dent J* 48:39-42.

Hughes T, Bockmann M, Mihailidis S, Bennett C, Harris A, Seow WK, et al. (2013). Genetic, epigenetic, and environmental influences on dentofacial structures and oral health: ongoing studies of Australian twins and their families. *Twin Res Hum Genet* 16:43-51.

Hughes TE, Townsend GC, Pinkerton SK, Bockmann MR, Seow WK, Brook AH, et al. (2014). The teeth and faces of twins: providing insights into dentofacial development and oral health for practising oral health professionals. *Aust Dent J* 59 (1 Suppl):101-116.

Townsend G, Bockmann M, Hughes T, Mihailidis S, Seow WK, Brook A (2012). New approaches to dental anthropology based on the study of twins. In: *New Directions in Dental Anthropology: paradigms, methodologies and outcomes.* Townsend G, Kanazawa E, Takayama H, editors. Adelaide: University of Adelaide Press, pp. 10-21.

Williams SD, Hughes TE, Adler CJ, Brook AH, Townsend GC (2014). Epigenetics: a new frontier in dentistry. *Aust Dent J* 59 (1 Suppl):23-33.

Woodroffe S, Mihailidis S, Hughes T, Bockmann M, Seow WK, Gotjamanos T, et al. (2010). Primary tooth emergence in Australian children: timing, sequence and patterns of asymmetry. *Aust Dent J* 55:245-251.

Yong R, Ranjitkar S, Townsend GC, Smith RN, Evans AR, Hughes TE, et al. (2014). Dental phenomics: advancing genotype to phenotype correlations in craniofacial research. *Aust Dent J* 59 (1 Suppl):34-47.

Chapter Two

A HISTORICAL PERSPECTIVE

INTRODUCTION

The birth of twins has been of interest throughout human history. From the earliest recorded times a multiple birth generated considerable attention both within and outside the family. The fact that these offspring often shared the same physical characteristics led to many explanations about the possible underlying causes. These explanations often related more to the depth of the imagination than to any factual evidence. Without knowing the complexities of the twinning process, early societies had to construct explanations that ordinary people could understand and accept, and it is not surprising that many of these explanations were centred on the mythical aspects of their cultures and religions.

Attitudes toward twins and twinning varied considerably in different parts of the world and could change quite dramatically over time. In pre-industrial societies there appeared to be two distinct attitudes towards them. One linked more to the unexplained (mythological) supernatural aspect and the other to the practicality of living with twins. The lives of twins depended on their cultural acceptance by society. If they were seen as freaks of nature, then some societies would have no compunction in killing them, and this occurred widely throughout history. Reasons for killing twins varied, but most concerned the idea that twin creation went against the laws of nature. One example of this may be seen in the belief that it was 'animal-like' for a mother to produce two children at the same time, or that to have given birth to two babies must mean two fathers. Other beliefs likened twinning to the practice of adultery or even the involvement of an evil spirit, which could well have decided the fate of twins (Bryan, 1983).

The practicality of living with twins was also an important factor in determining how they were treated, particularly in nomadic societies where it became almost impossible to breastfeed two babies when food was scarce and the population was continually on the move to find food and water. In contrast, other societies accepted and even welcomed twins if, for example, the chief of a tribe had twins and the tribe then prospered. If the birth of twins coincided with 'good omens', then the likelihood of good fortune would normally be associated with them.

One of the difficulties confronting those who developed and dictated the laws of a particular society arose when providing some form of explanation as to why twins should be accepted or not. Many early interpretations represented a fusion or balance between mythology or fantasy and reality or the truths of everyday life. When it came to rearing twins, ordinary people probably had more down-to-earth views, not the least being that they had two more mouths to feed rather than one. It seems that when it became necessary for any early society to explain the twinning process to its people, the explanation tended to incorporate mystery with the practicality of the known world.

Mythological beginnings

In one of the earliest recordings of twins found in the Pantheon of Ancient Mesopotamia, it is noted that the twin divinities Lugalgirra and Meslamtaea were interpreted as godlike beings, as indeed were the twins recorded in both the Babylon and Assyrian civilizations (Gedda, 1961). In these early references, twins were endowed with supernatural powers but had little influence over the everyday lives of the people. With the discovery of the Vedic Sanskrit Hindu texts of Ancient India, it was noted that the god-like twins referred to as Asvins adopted the occupation of medical practitioners with the power to heal and reverse the ageing process through the medium of prayer.

By reading these selected early twin references it is possible to see the development of explanations about twinning and twins from the purely supernatural to something that could be recognised and understood more by ordinary people. This incorporation of human values into twin mythology provided much greater meaning and understanding of their existence within their respective societies. Unlike so many other mythical stories and beliefs, the tangible presence of twins required more than parental acceptance; it required societies to accept them as being different. If society did not approve, then the parents of twins faced ostracism and they had to decide whether they were prepared to live with their twins or not.

A historical perspective

Because many twins were noted to be similar in appearance, the idea of twin inseparability emerged. Some beliefs included the notion that twins were two people with a single mind, and that they would be incapable of surviving unless they stayed together. This was a belief fostered in the Greek myth of the twins Castor and Pollux. When Castor was killed in battle, Pollux pleaded with his father, Zeus, to be reunited with his dead brother. His wish was granted and both brothers were installed as twin stars in the constellation of Gemini. Elizabeth Bryan, in her book *The Nature and Nurture of Twins*, uses the myth of Narcissus to further illustrate twin inseparability. She explains that when Narcissus's twin sister died, he spent many hours looking at his reflection in a pool, not to admire his own image, but to be reminded always of hers (Bryan, 1983).

Not all interactions between twins were harmonious. The myth of Romulus and Remus, whilst accentuating twin sharing (both twins having been suckled by a she-wolf), developed the theme of competition, culminating in the death of Remus over a dispute with Romulus about where the city of Rome should be built (Figure 2.1).

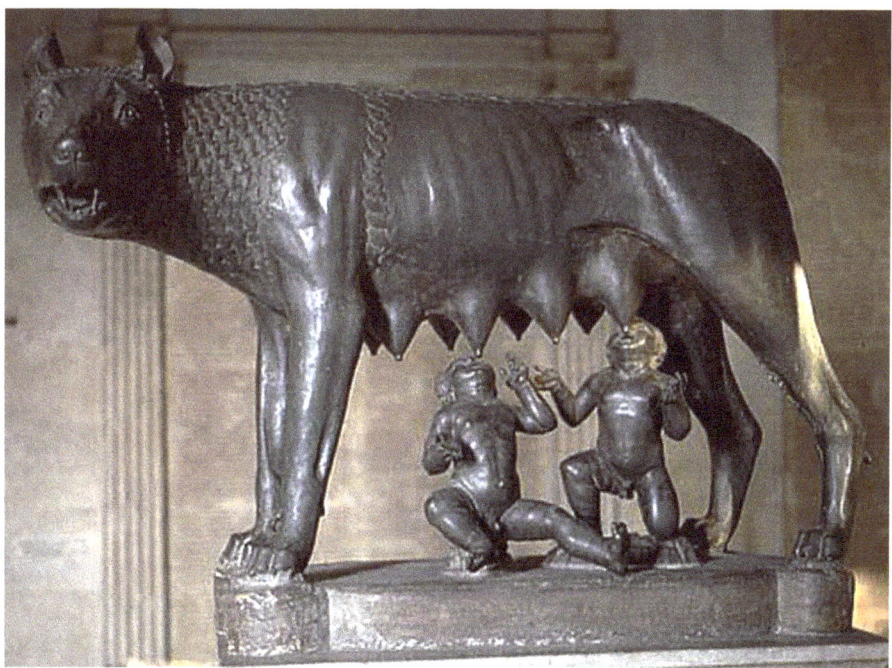

Figure 2.1
The statue of Romulus and Remus in the Palazzo dei Conservatori, Capitolini Musie, Rome. Photograph courtesy of Geraldine Yam.

Romulus was attributed with the virtues of courage, strength and purpose, and it was imperative to the Roman mentality that these attributes should predominate and be inculcated in the founder. Competition also governed the actions of the biblical twins Esau and Jacob in their struggle for recognition of first birthright.

Twins in the Theatre

With the advent of theatre and literature, new dimensions were created whereby the perception of twins became less concerned with myth and superstition and more with the idea that twins were normal human beings. Whether by travelling players or by the conventional theatre, it became possible to produce works that emphasised the involvement of twins in everyday life.

One of the earliest of these plays was the *Menaechmi*. Thought to have been composed in Sicily by Epicharmus in the fifth century BC, this play developed plots concerning twin resemblance, separation, confusion and comedy. The central theme in these works — and also the works of the sixteenth-century playwrights Gian Giorgio Trissino, Agnolo Firenzuola and Juan de Timoneda — was the farce of mistaken identity. These plays were written before William Shakespeare wrote his twin-inspired comedy plays, *The Comedy of Errors* (probably written between 1589 and 1595) and *Twelfth Night or What You Will* (probably written between 1600 and 1602).

These plays, perhaps more than any other means of communication, informed the populace about what it was like to be a twin and about the problems twins faced in the world. In these plays the previous supernatural concepts associated with twins were replaced by an observed twin lifestyle, with comedy often being the predominant theme (Figure 2.2).

Shakespeare, himself the father of twins (Hamnet and Judith), emphasised, whether knowingly or not, the concept that twinship need not necessarily be an entirely male preserve. *Twelfth Night* has a male/female format with the different-sex twins being developed in the male leading roles. Shakespeare's development of the character Viola places an emphasis on female involvement in affairs central to the theme of the play (diplomatic negotiation). The development of the male/female twin combination in this play may well have been the result of Shakespeare's experience as a father of a different-sex twin pair. What is particularly interesting is how both the male and female characters are mistaken for each other: 'one face, one voice, one

A historical perspective

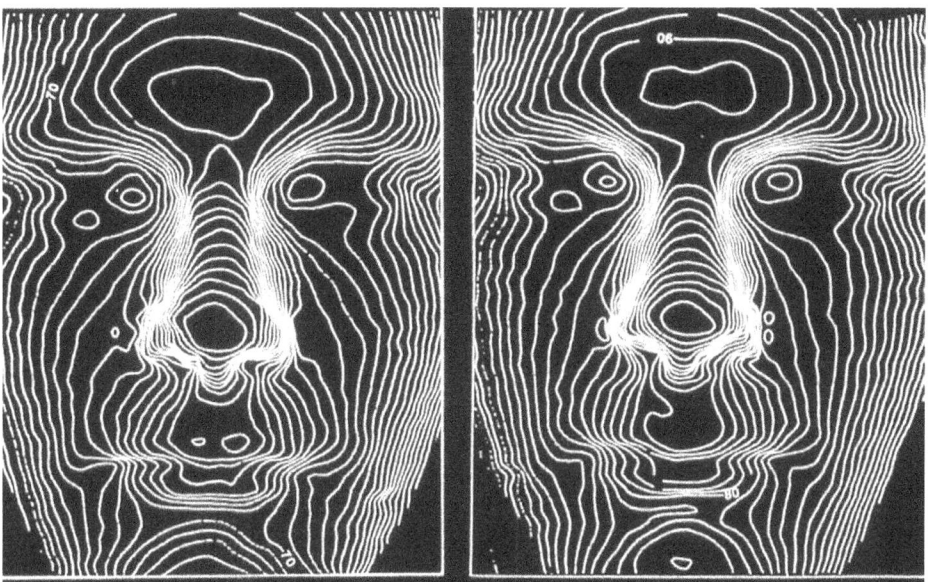

Figure 2.2
These facial contour maps of a pair of twins from one of our studies were used in the program for *The Comedy of Errors*, a State Theatre Company presentation at the Festival Theatre, Adelaide, during the 1990s.

habit and two persons'. It raises an interesting question: how masculine did Viola appear to the other characters in the play, and also to the audience? Or how feminine in appearance was Sebastian?

Twins became effective characters in theatrical productions because playwrights could bring together the very attributes that made them interesting to ordinary people. Their similarities and their differences could be developed and used to create situations which highlighted the thoughts and feelings we all experience in facing the problems of everyday life. While theatre opened people's minds to what it was like to be a twin, it could not expand that understanding to the same extent that literature, in the form of a novel, could.

Twins in literature

One example of the inclusion of twins in novels is the development of fear and prejudice experienced by twins in George Sand's nineteenth-century novel *La petite*

Fadette. Sand uses a family situation to develop the concept of twin separation being allied to obsession. The difference in parental attitudes over the rearing of the twin boys, with the father's interests becoming paramount, leads to conflict which results in tragedy (Sand, 1849). Another interesting study of the relationship between twins is provided in Thornton Wilder's classic novel *The Bridge of San Luis Rey*. In this book, Wilder (himself a twin survivor whose twin brother died at birth) explores the theme of twin compatibility and loss. Brought up as orphans, Esteban and Manuel live their lives isolated from the world around them.

Wilder (1927) described his twins in these words:

Because they had no family, because they were twins, and because they were brought up by women, they were silent. There was in them a curious shame in regard to their resemblance. They had to live in a world where it was the subject of continual comment and joking. It was never funny to them and they suffered the eternal pleasantries with stolid patience.

Their isolation was so complete that little was allowed to penetrate their self-imposed insulation from society. The only thing that did was Manuel's love for Camila, and the way his unrequited love threatened the world they had made for themselves. With the death of Manuel and the consequent remorse of Esteban, the collapse of the bridge at San Luis Rey united the twins in death.

Sand's and Wilder's novels, written 100 years apart, share the similar theme of twin unrest caused by external pressures imposed by the societies in which they lived, and over which they had little control. What was important to both sets of twins and to the plots of both novels was the unreasonable attitudes of the communities in which the twins lived. In both instances society had great difficulty in accepting that each member of a twin pair needed to be seen and treated as an individual with control over his or her own life. The other characteristic of twins emphasised in these novels was the bonding between co-twins and how that bonding affected their behaviour. The more the twins behaved and acted as one person, the more society reacted against them. Such cause and effect supports the notion of ESP (extra sensory perception), in that it became a way in which society attempted to explain why twins could converse with each other in ways that nobody else could understand.

The notion that twins should be seen as being 'naturally' different from other people was challenged in Aldous Huxley's *Brave New World* (1932). In this book Huxley created a totalitarian world populated with genetically engineered clones. Each member was produced from the same gene pool and subjected to different oxygen levels during development. The higher the levels of oxygen given to individuals, the more intelligent they became and, conversely, the lower the levels, the less intelligent the individual. Each person was subjected to conditioning programmes designed to create a society in which every member was designed to perform specific tasks and to want nothing more than to perform those tasks for the sake of the society. Society in Huxley's world was based upon unnatural stability supported by conditioned contentment. *Brave New World* removed entirely the distinction between twins and singletons — and with it every accepted notion that might set them apart.

TWINS IN SCIENCE

From a historical viewpoint, the scientific interpretations of twins and twinning differed considerably from interpretations made by non-scientific commentators. Perhaps the biggest difference was that the scientific approach considered that the twinning process could be explained within the context of medical knowledge, not in terms of myths or unsubstantiated beliefs. Many of the early scientific theories relating to the twinning process arose in Ancient Greece between 500 and 350 BC. This was a period when philosophers tried to separate fact from superstition, with the study of natural sciences holding a pre-eminent position in their thoughts. Hippocrates of Kos was one thinker who believed that twin births were caused by the sperm dividing into two sections, with each section impregnating one of the two uterine horns (Gedda, 1961). He also reasoned that conjoined twins were created when there was excessive sperm produced — more than enough for one child, but not enough for two.

If there was one guiding principle in these philosophers' thinking, it appears to be that everything that occurred in nature must have a reason. Empedocles was another who believed that an excess of sperm was the cause of twins. He also thought that excessive heat in the uterus could possibly divide the sperm, leading to more than one individual being formed. Democritus of Abdera, originator of the atomic theory, considered that acts of sexual intercourse performed within relatively short periods of time enabled the sperm to produce more than one embryo (Gedda, 1961).

Aristotle also considered the issue of twin births, but, instead of limiting his considerations to the action of sperm alone, he developed ideas relating to the phenomenon of co-development. His theories were based upon the multiparous nature of animal births and, in particular, the often observed conjoined monstrosities which accompanied such births. Evidence from animal studies convinced him that two or more separate embryos were normally created, which would produce separate individuals if allowed to remain apart. However, if through some unknown cause they were allowed to come into contact with each other they would fuse and form a monstrosity. The degree of fusion was relative to the degree of contact. Should two or more embryos be created without contacting each other, then Aristotle favoured Democritus's concept of the twinning process (Gedda, 1961).

It could be argued that through his association of ideas Aristotle had opened up the possibilities for future researchers to develop new notions about how twins were formed. This linking of research between human and animal twin studies could well have been the foundation for the discipline of teratology. This subject was popularised in the seventeenth century, and referred at that time to any observations of the physically abnormal; in the eighteenth century it was considered as the study of biological deformation; and in the twentieth century the term teratology was used to refer to the study of congenital malformations.

During Roman times there appears to have been little work done to either support or to refute the Greek theories of multiple births. Galen of Pergamon, like other eminent medical practitioners of the day, whilst specialising in medical theory and practice and having an interest in human reproduction and foetal development, was not known for any notable interest in the twinning process. Gaius Plinius Secundas — better known as Pliny the Elder, author of *The Natural History* — devoted much of his time to the reporting of multiple births, but he offered little or no explanation as to the reasons behind their formation (Gedda, 1961). These Roman men of science and medicine set the stage for future research, with less emphasis being placed on the theoretical view of the twinning process and more on the obstetrical problems associated with it.

Between the eighth and thirteenth centuries, the Arabic and the Salernitan schools of medicine were held in high regard and did much to promote medical knowledge; but they seem to have done little more than repeat the observations of twins made in the past. It was in the Renaissance Period that significant developments occurred, enabling twin research to advance in ways it had never done before. These developments centred upon the revival of the ideas of Greek, Roman and Arabic medical scientists, the advent of the written word, and the ability to read translations of the works of past and present men of science. Of the past medical commentators, Hippocrates, Aristotle and Galen became important to the Renaissance scientists — the former two because of their comments relating to the phenomenon of conjoined twins, and the latter because of his book *Spiritus Animalis*, of which 500 English translation editions were printed between 1490 and 1538 (Snow-Smith, 2004).

Jacob Locher (1499) produced one of the first printed illustrations of conjoined twins, and Ambroise Paré (1575) attempted to explain the different types of conjoined twins in terms that everyone could understand. He thought that constriction of the womb — whether through external or internal pressure, as in muscle constriction or tight clothing — was a prime cause of conjoined twins or monstrosities. This view of conjoined twins as being monstrosities was common throughout much of this period and beyond, and those conjoined twins who survived became objects of study or curiosity. Drawings of conjoined twins appeared in scientific publications — for example, Fortunio Liceti's *De monstrorum caussis, natura, et differentiis libri duo* (1634) — and twins also often appeared in sideshows, being depicted as freaks of nature (Bondeson, 1993).

There have been other issues that have made people think differently about twins. In the seventeenth and eighteenth centuries, the phenomenon of conjoined twinning caught the public's attention through the medium of published pamphlets. These popular publications were known in England as 'Monster' Broadsides, and they were used to exploit the 'sensational'. Conjoined-twin births fell into that category because they enabled the authors to emphasise, in every lurid detail, the birth of conjoined twins. In one of these pamphlets, conjoined twins appeared as a 'monstrous work of Nature' and, besides describing their physical appearance, the author (an unknown gentleman of Taunton Deane in Somerset) went to great lengths to outline the religious implications of their birth (Anon, 1680).

Publicity of this nature was both good and bad for the parents of conjoined children. It was good in the sense that, through the interest generated by the pamphlet, many people thronged to view the twins and purchased mementos of their visit, thus generating income to provide for the twins' future welfare. It was bad in the sense that society often viewed these children as portents of impending evil, a belief common in the period 1600-1800 when ordinary people attempted to understand the inexplicable.

Galen's work was one of several medical textbooks that were referred to extensively during the Renaissance period (Snow-Smith, 2004). The value of his work was its ability to inform and inspire the work of others. Perhaps the greatest of Galen's readers was Leonardo da Vinci. With past knowledge affecting Renaissance thinking, it was not surprising that there was a blending of art and science during this time in attempts to further knowledge relating to the human body. Sculptors, such as Carlo Mondini of Bolongna, prepared wax depictions of dichorionic and monochorionic twins in the uterus. These depictions were not only works of art but also accurate representations of the anatomy of twins within the womb. As more books were published and people became literate, further artistic representations were made that were based on direct obstetrical observations. These representations could be formed from metal (copper) engravings or woodcuts, and were predominantly designed for use in conjunction with medically inspired literature.

Leonardo da Vinci, above all others of his time, was instrumental in integrating the transcription of anatomical observations with direct anatomical dissections. The collection of notes and sketches in his 'Treatise on Anatomy', whilst highlighting his anatomical knowledge and artistic ability, did not impact upon those who shared his medical interests, to the degree that the 'Treatise' only came to light 300 years after his death. When it did, it set new standards in anatomical depiction, and da Vinci could well be thought of as the originator of scientific illustration (Snow-Smith, 2004).

The seventeenth century saw important advances in several key areas of medicine. One area was the description of a form of twinning which was characterised by twins occupying a common amniotic sac (monoamniotic twin pregnancy). According to Ferdinand Pauls (1969):

> [t]he first comprehensive review of the literature on monoamniotic twinning was made in 1935 by Quigley, who found 109 cases. The next review by Raphael in 1961 added a further 74 cases, bringing the total reported in the world literature to 183.

This observation illustrates the fact that many years were to pass between the discovery of a twinning phenomenon and reports being made about its frequency.

One interesting fact about conjoined twins was that, despite the problems associated with their physical deformities and the limited surgical knowledge at the time, the first recorded successful separation of conjoined twins was made by Johannes Fatio in 1689 (Kompanje, 2004). Meanwhile, another problem associated with conjoined twins was: how could the mother survive the trauma of such a birth? For example, how many required caesarean deliveries? It must be assumed that the circumstances surrounding such a delivery were different in every case, making reporting of conjoined-twin births very difficult.

In the eighteenth century, studies of the twinning process did not seem to dominate the minds of the great medical and scientific people of the day. Obstetrics, surgery and anatomical dissection were the prime topics for research, with Johann Friedrich Meckel the Younger, John Hunter and William Smellie making their names in these fields. Although they did not concentrate directly on building knowledge about twins and twinning, these men did contribute to related areas, including teratology and obstetrics.

Meckel, famous for his discovery of the diverticulum (an abnormal pouch or sac opening from a hollow organ such as the colon or bladder), also made an impressive contribution to understanding abnormalities during embryological development. He made the first comprehensive and analytical description of birth defects. When consideration is given to the association of birth defects, multiple births and the conjoined 'monstrosity' syndrome, his work stands out as not being influenced by fantasy or morality. One of the greatest pathologists and anatomists of his day, John Hunter, added to the knowledge of twinning by his dissections of freemartins. These are normally associated with twin births in cattle, in which the female of the twin pair does not breed or give milk. Through his dissections he detected that a freemartin always had a male twin (Hunter, 1779).

Meckel and Hunter were primarily anatomists, while William Smellie was a leader in obstetrics. His contribution to medical science concerned the theoretical basis and practice of childbirth. He based both his teaching and practice upon scientific principles, and he created a set of anatomical tables which were designed to provide detailed explanations of most aspects of midwifery. These men applied science to their respective research interests, and were instrumental in establishing methods which those who followed could emulate. In particular, they laid the foundations of a scientific approach to solving problems, medical or otherwise, which so characterised the nineteenth century.

Perhaps the most well-known and publicised conjoined twins in history were Chang and Eng. Born in Siam in 1811, they became famous as public exhibits travelling from Siam to America and England (Figure 2.3). As showground curiosities they were billed as 'The Siamese Double Boys'. Joined at the lower chest, they also became subjects for medical examinations aiming to discover the key structures which

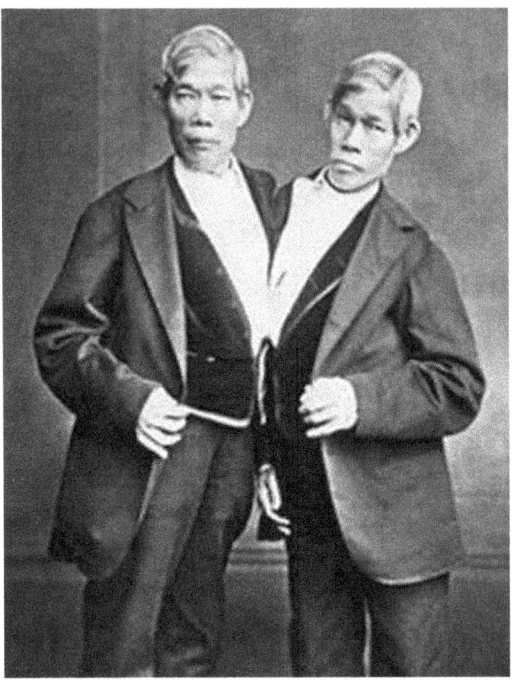

Figure 2.3
Chang and Eng Bunker in later life.
http://dc.lib.unc.edu/cdm/singleitem/collection/bunkers/id/376/rec/1

joined them together. They were very popular with the public, and they were feted wherever they went. Returning to America in 1832, they became naturalised citizens and eventually married, having twenty-one children between them. Chang died on 17 January 1874 and a few hours later Eng also died. Their importance to the way society viewed conjoined twins was dramatic.

Chang and Eng, through their popularity, made people aware of the problems suffered by conjoined twins. Their condition proved that their physical handicap did not mean they could not live normal lives. It was also through their Asian origin that the term 'Siamese twins' became associated with conjoined twins in general.

THE CONCEPT OF NATURE VERSUS NURTURE

It was not until the nineteenth century that the relationship between human individuality and the environment in which that individuality developed was seriously

A historical perspective

researched. The Age of Enlightenment provided the necessary conditions for those promoting human knowledge to have both a belief in the essence of nature, and a devotion to understanding human development. From the point of view of twins, these beliefs led to scientific debate about nature versus nurture. A leading figure in this debate was Sir Francis Galton (Figure 2.4). He expressed his understanding of the phrase in these words:

> The phrase 'nature versus nurture' is a convenient jingle of words, for it separates under two distinct heads the innumerable elements of which personality is composed. Nature is all that a man brings with himself into the world; nurture is every influence from without that affects him after his birth. The distinction is clear: the one produces the infant such as it actually is, including its latent faculties of growth of body and mind; the other affords the environment amid which growth takes place, by which natural tendencies may be strengthened or thwarted, or wholly new ones implanted. (Galton, 1874)

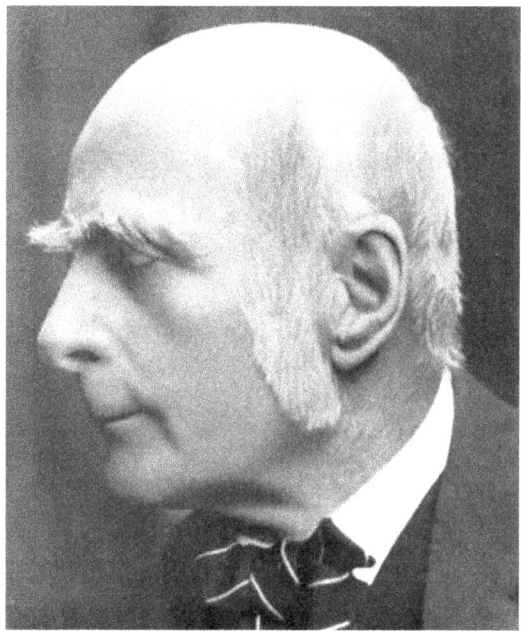

Figure 2.4
Sir Francis Galton, photographed circa 1870.
Courtesy of Gavan Tredoux, site editor http://galton.org/

Galton was influenced in his thinking by the publication of Charles Darwin's *On the Origin of Species* (1859), particularly Darwin's comments on the observed variation associated with the breeding of animals. The study of human variation became a central theme in Galton's work. According to David Burbridge (2001), Galton's primary studies regarding twins began in November 1874. He was interested in establishing whether the differences observed in human intelligence could be attributed to hereditary ('nature') or to environmental ('nurture') factors.

One method Galton used to determine the contributions of 'nature and nurture' to observed similarities and differences between twins was to provide a questionnaire to 190 fellows of the Royal Society. His intention in using this survey was to see whether the intelligence exhibited by the fellows was acquired through inheritance or predominantly through environmental influences. In other words, was their interest in science innate or had it developed through their upbringing? He was also interested in finding out whether there was evidence of twin births in the family histories of the fellows in his sample, and whether they would agree to pass his questionnaire to other contacts who were twins or who were related to twins. The results of this research were published in 1874 in a book entitled *English Men of Science: Their Nature and Nurture*. Galton felt that his results did show that a level of intelligence was inherited, but his findings were inconclusive in determining how much variation could be attributed to 'nature' over 'nurture'.

Realising that his study was limited, Galton designed a more specific programme which concentrated on twin comparisons. Questions were devised that concerned twins who appeared alike at birth but were placed into totally different environments, and twins who were unlike each other at birth but placed into similar environments. Following the format of his earlier questionnaire, Galton sought details on the strength of resemblance between twins, including features such as height, weight, fit of clothes, hair and eye colour, athletic abilities, manual skills, handwriting, tone of voice, tastes, disposition and health. He also asked the twins about their education and subsequent pursuits, the extent to which their similarity had decreased with age, and their own assessment of why this may have occurred (Burbridge, 2001).

What is important to note is that Galton, at this time, had decided on a method of study in which a hypothesis was formed and then the data obtained were used to test that hypothesis. In other words, he structured what later became known as a 'method' or 'model' of twin research — a specific method of research involving comparisons within and between pairs of twins.

His conclusion, published under the title *The History of Twins* (Galton, 1875), echoed the findings of his 1874 paper, which concluded that when consideration was given to the degrees of similarity, twins generally exhibited moderate forms of similarity to each other, but that more extremes of similarity or dissimilarity were noted in those twins who were of the same sex. This observation reinforced the idea that 'nature' had more input upon twin formation than 'nurture'. It also emphasised the point that when it came to distinguishing physical characteristics within a collection of twin data, it was easier to define and categorise similarity in a more organised way. Burbridge (2001) makes the observation:

> The modern reader may assume that Galton is here recognizing the distinction between monozygotic (identical) and dizygotic (fraternal) twins … Galton was indeed aware that some twins were produced from a single egg, while others came from separate eggs.

In the mid-1870s there was considerable debate amongst researchers in Europe and America over the questions of human embryo separation and methods of fertilisation. It was not possible for Galton or anyone else at this time to definitely state that twins received identical genetic material from a single fertilised egg. They simply did not know the complexities involved in the formation of monozygotic (so-called identical) and dizygotic (so-called non-identical) twins.

What is also important in Galton's approach to research was that he was quite willing to change his conceptions as more facts came to light. For example, he recognised the extensive influence of 'nurture' during the stages of human development, from conception to the onset of birth, not just the environment after birth (Galton, 1883). He also recognised that in asking questions about dissimilarity he might have created a bias through encouraging exaggerated responses from his subjects. Galton, therefore, established two fundamental principles of modern research — the willingness to change research goals once evidence demands a change, and also the need to consider factors that may create bias or lead to unexpected outcomes.

The question of who actually proposed the 'twin method' is controversial. Richard Rende and colleagues (1990) make the point that

> … Galton's delight in discovering twins was to assess the ability of the environment to make initially similar twins different and to make initially

different twins similar. Galton thought that all of his twins — both the similar and the dissimilar pairs — were one-egg twins, what we now call identical twins. He did not suggest comparing one-egg and two-egg twins. Thus, it is not correct to claim that Galton proposed the twin method.

Rende and colleagues further state that no other studies concerning twin resemblance were published until Edward Thorndike (1905) wrote a paper concerning twin mental and physical resemblance, relating that resemblance to a series of carefully designed cognitive tests. It was not until twenty years later (fifty years after Galton) that Curtis Merriman (1924) wrote a paper entitled *The Intellectual Resemblance of Twins* in which he noted that there was a difference between identical and non-identical twins. Whilst he did not follow up this observation, he had made an important distinction between the differing twin groups.

According to Rende and colleagues, the first authors who actually compared the correlations of monozygotic and dizygotic twins for IQ (intelligence quotient) were Gladys Tallman (1928) and Alex Wingfield and Peter Sandiford (1928). Rende and colleagues also emphasised that the twin model could be attributed to the joint discoveries of Curtis Merriman and Hermann Siemens in the 1920s. However, Oliver Mayo (2009) noted that the twin model could not be developed into a single identifiable entity until three distinct evolutionary stages of research had been accomplished:

> ... a proper understanding of the difference between MZ and DZ twins, which was barely achieved by the end of 19th century; a clearly understood and correct model for inheritance, which was 'rediscovered' around 1900; and a clear method for causal assignment of variability, which Fisher achieved in 1918.

Mayo further makes the point that between the years 1900 to the mid-1920s there were discoveries made by researchers which, whilst not covering all of the above three requirements, addressed one or two of them. Examples given are Kristine Bonnevie (1924) and Hermann Siemens (1924), who reached similar conclusions that monozygotic and dizygotic twins needed to be properly diagnosed. Once this difference was established it was possible to construct correlations within the twin pairs. With regard to the first and second requirements, Mayo felt that Wilhelm Weinberg (1901) and Heinrich Poll (1914) had adequately satisfied these components of the twin model.

What makes Poll an important figure in the decades before the First World War was his ability to think of identical twin pairs as subjects who could be used in research involving genetics. According to Mayo (2009), Poll noted that

A historical perspective

> MZ twins and triplets are in fact the sole humans with identical genomes, the sole isozygotic individuals: for the same sperm and the same egg should yield them the same genetical endowment, according to theory. (Poll, 1914)

Such a concept made him a pioneer of twin studies and genetic research. He was able to show that fingerprints of twins could be used as genetic markers and, as such, could be used in studies concerning similarity and dissimilarity, and even in determining cases of paternity. Above all, Poll proposed the idea that monozygotic twin pairs could be used as a type of control group whose variability would indicate environmental differences unaffected by genetic differences.

From a historical perspective, Poll's life had several fascinating aspects (Braund and Sutton, 2008). One was that so much of his work in the early 1900s was in German and, either through difficulty in translation or availability, was not widely known. Other issues relate to the First World War and its anti-German aftermath. Above all, however, it was his interest in eugenics and his belief in the state having control over human reproductive behaviour which may have condemned his later work to relative obscurity.

In the period under discussion, meanwhile, Hermann Siemens wrote a book primarily concerned with psychological and skin disorders. Siemens emphasised skin disorders in this work, and, importantly, considered comparisons in both identical and non-identical twins. His purpose was to judge the hereditary influence on both body features and the intellectual performance of his subjects (Siemens, 1924). Also in this decade, the Swedish eugenist and statistician Gunnar Dahlberg designed a statistical method that allowed measurement error to be quantified. He was one of the first to demonstrate the value of studying twins as well (Dahlberg, 1926).

INHERITANCE AND MENDELIAN GENETICS

Allied to Darwin's theory of natural selection and to Jean-Baptiste Lamarck's thoughts on evolution, complex questions concerning the mechanisms of inheritance were also being considered at this time. Although never directly linked to twin research, the discovery of how one organism can pass certain characteristics to its offspring was to play an important part in the future understanding of the development of twins. Jean-Baptiste Lamarck had devised a theory of evolution which encompassed two distinct ideas concerning how organisms, during their lifetime, pass certain information to their offspring. He considered that if an animal constantly used part of its body to achieve an outcome, then that part of its body would develop accordingly. Conversely, any part of an animal's body which was not used would weaken and deteriorate. These 'modifications' would then be passed on to the offspring of the animal and therefore, over time — as needs changed and behaviours changed — there would be a gradual transmutation of the animal species (Lamarck, 1809). It is fascinating to note how recent discoveries in the field of epigenetics have reignited interest in Lamarckian evolution.

Charles Darwin (1859) also favoured the idea of inheritance of acquired factors in his concept of continuous evolution. He developed the theory of 'pangenesis', which assumed that cells could create tiny particles, or so-called pangenes or gemmules as he termed them, and these would contain information concerning the parent. This information would diffuse and collect in the reproductive organs, and therefore be passed from parent to offspring. With the acquisition of knowledge about the way genetic expression passes information from one generation to the next, Darwin's ideas were seen to be flawed. It was not until the work of Gregor Johann Mendel that the biological laws governing the passage of information from one generation to the next were discovered (Figure 2.5).

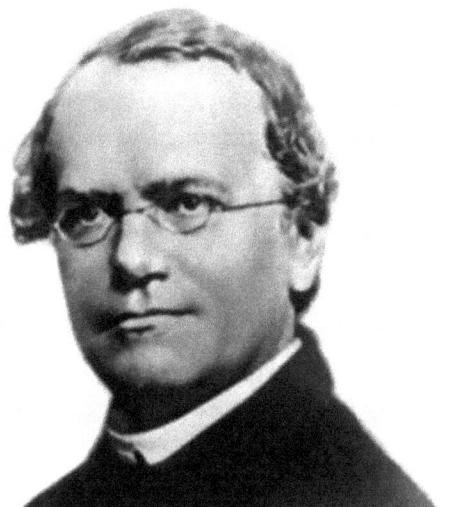

Figure 2.5
Gregor Johann Mendel (1822-1884).
http://commons.wikimedia.org/wiki/File:Gregor_Mendel.jpg

A historical perspective

Gregor Johann Mendel developed a research programme to discover how information was passed from parents to offspring. In 1843, after a concentrated period of time studying philosophy and physics at the Olmutz Philosophical Institute, he entered an Augustinian monastery (the Abbey of St Thomas in Brno, Czechoslovakia). It was at this monastery that he conducted his experiments on plants that earned him the title of 'the father of genetics'.

Many of his experiments were conducted using the pea species *Pisum sativum*, and were designed to discover hereditary traits of plants. By studying generations of pea specimens, Mendel was able to confirm that pea offspring retained the essential traits of the parental plants and were not influenced by their environment. He studied several pea plant traits: flower colour, position, length, seed colour, pod shape and pod colour. His observations were explained in two principles: the principle of segregation and the principle of independent assortment. These principles later became known as Mendel's Laws of Inheritance. It was not until 1900 that Mendel's work was 'rediscovered' by the scientific community and its implications were considered in relation to Darwin's concepts of evolution and natural selection.

TWIN RESEARCH: A QUESTION OF ETHICS

The 'nature' (hereditary) versus 'nurture' (environmental) question was to continue for much of the first half of the twentieth century. With growing understanding of genetic theory, studies of twins became more sophisticated. One infamous phase of twin research concerned the study of psychology and eugenics. Based upon the work of Kurt Gottschaldt, who used twins to explain observed psychological traits and patterns of behaviour, research emerged that was governed more by political ideology and less by scientific enquiry. Fostered by the political ideology of Nazi Germany and its belief in the creation of a pure-bred Aryan race, Heinrich Himmler gave permission for Otmar Freiherr von Verschuer, who was then working at the Kaiser Wilhelm Institute, to conduct research designed to uncover the secrets of heredity.

Working under von Verschuer's direction, Joseph Mengele conducted experiments on twins in the concentration camp at Auschwitz in Poland during World War II. These experiments involved blood transfusions from one twin to another, eye operations to induce blindness, pain induction and injections of disease-causing organisms. In cases of experimentation leading to death, detailed autopsies were also performed. All these experiments on twin subjects were designed to examine what made them different from singletons and how understanding these differences could benefit the German race. It was thought that an understanding of genetics could enable desirable human features to be developed (positive eugenics) and that this would lead to the creation of a pure race. It was appreciated that not every gene expression was desirable, and this gave rise to the concept of negative eugenics — that is, the 'improvement' of human populations by removal of deleterious genes.

The 'research' practised by Mengele raised the issue of ethical experimentation, and the question of what is acceptable, and what is not, in scientific discovery. To Mengele and his associates, the end justified the means. Today, the involvement of human subjects in scientific experimentation is governed by ethical values and strict rules designed to safeguard the rights of participants. Our modern codes of scientific ethical behaviour can trace their origins to the Judgement of Nuremberg (1947) in which ten ethical standards were designed to form a foundation upon which future principles could be applied, followed by The Declaration of Helsinki (1964), which both strengthened the existing regulations and broadened their scope.

In Australia, the 'National Statement on Ethical Conduct in Research Involving Humans' (2007) contains guidelines for ethical conduct in scientific research which are in accordance with the National Health and Medical Research Council Act 1992. However, consideration of ethical values should not be restricted to human experiments which involve direct contact with participants. They are also important in the actual conduct of the research itself. One example of what could be called 'unethical practice' has been associated with the research of Sir Cyril Burt. Burt, an educational psychologist, published a series of papers which concerned the genetics of intelligence. Burt argued that heredity (nature) had a greater impact upon intellectual ability than that generated by the environment (nurture). The accusations made against Burt were based on certain anomalies researchers noted in the values of correlation coefficients he reported between his monozygotic twin subjects for IQ scores. Debate ensued as to whether Burt's findings were generated through inexcusable carelessness or by conscious fakery. According to Stephen J Gould in his chapter 'The Real Error of Cyril Burt' it was a deliberate attempt on Burt's part to falsify his data (Gould, 1981).

A historical perspective

Twin research: specialisation

It was in the 1920s and 1930s that twin research reached a level in which specialised areas could be identified. Studies concerning twin resemblance, age, identity, intelligence and handedness became areas of interest.

Some of the questions posed included: Does age have any bearing on resemblance in twins? Do like-sex twin pairs show a greater degree of resemblance than unlike-sex twin pairs? Do twins in general show a greater degree of resemblance than other family siblings? (Lauterbach, 1925). These questions illustrate that research was attempting to explain observable differences in twins and to link these differences to a (genetic) hereditary cause rather than to environmental ones. Another leading question asked at this time was: 'How great is the probability that, in a given trait, one-egg twins are not alike? and: how great is the probability that (in the same trait) two-egg twins are alike?' (Siemens, 1927). Such ideas reinforced the concept that studies involving the determination of trait expression and frequency in twin pairs should concentrate more upon hereditary factors than environmental ones.

Intelligence testing between monozygotic and dizygotic twin pairs was also attempted and, although the results were inconclusive, there was some evidence to support the view that the IQ was higher in the monozygotic groups and lower in dizygotic twins, with the lowest values being in the unlike-sex dizygotic pairs (Wingfield and Sandiford, 1928).

In the 1930s two further twin studies were developed. These were studies of handedness and an investigation of monozygotic twins reared apart. It had been noticed by Wilhelm Weitz (1924), Gunnar Dahlberg (1926) and Horatio Newman (1928a,b) that identical twins displayed a greater percentage of left-handedness than fraternal twins. Ideas were developed in an attempt to explain why such handedness occurred. Often these explanations related to the observed effect of higher levels of reversed asymmetry (mirror imaging) during development in monozygotic twins than in dizygotic twins (Wilson and Jones, 1932). The second twin study which emerged about this time was to consider the observed similarities and differences in monozygotic twins reared apart (Newman, 1934). Although much of this work was descriptive, its importance to future studies was that researchers placed greater emphasis upon environmental influences affecting individuals, rather than concentrating solely on genetic factors.

Twin Studies

TWIN RESEARCH: THE GREAT STEPS FORWARD

Perhaps the greatest discovery in the twentieth century, which revolutionised studies involving genetically inspired research, was the discovery of the molecular structure of deoxyribonucleic acid (DNA). Further details of the birth and development of the DNA theory of inheritance, which culminated in this discovery, have been provided recently by Petter Portin (2014).

Francis Crick and James Watson, working in Cambridge in 1953, announced to the world that they had discovered the structure of the deoxyribonucleic acid molecule and how genetic information was transferred between individuals via DNA. What this discovery meant to twin research was that more detailed tests for zygosity could be conducted based on comparisons of DNA. Accurate information about twin zygosities has enabled more sophisticated genetic models to be constructed, and has removed the problem which plagued previous research, where so much was based on assumption. Once it could be positively established that monozygotic co-twins shared the same genes and dizygotic co-twins only shared (on average) half their genes, it became possible to further extend the classical twin model in ways that 'pre-DNA-discovery' researchers could only dream about.

One of the most difficult problems facing researchers in the early twentieth century was to determine how inheritance influenced quantitative factors compared with qualitative ones. The term 'quantitative' usually describes continuously variable data, whereas data that are separated into distinct types or categories are thought of as 'qualitative'. Explanatory problems arose when attempts were made to interpret quantitative data describing individual differences based on the Galtonian model of inheritance. There were those who felt that Galton's data could best be expressed using Mendelian principles. A protégé of Galton was Karl Pearson, who formulated a statistical model to Galton's theory of inheritance (Pearson, 1904).

If this model lacked one essential ingredient, it was to establish a coherent account of how correlations between relatives could be explained. In 1910 Wilhelm Weinberg published a paper in which he had worked out ratios regarding these correlations between relatives in a randomly mating population. Using his statistical method, he proved that his results were consistent with Mendelian inheritance theory (Weinberg, 1910). He also worked out a method to determine the proportion of monozygotic and dizygotic twins from a sample of similar-sex twins at a time

A historical perspective

when the biological origin of the twin types was not fully understood. In addition, Weinberg considered phenotypic variation and segregated this variation into what he considered to be genetically inspired and environmental causes. From his work with twin data he came to the conclusion that the birth of dizygotic twins was influenced more by genetic factors than the birth of monozygotic twins (Weinberg, 1901).

It fell to RA Fisher (Figure 2.6) to provide a statistical model which illustrated that every observable human trait was caused by numbers of individual genes which were inherited in the same way as outlined in Mendel's laws (Fisher, 1936). This model later became known as a polygenic model. Fisher's statistical model, sometimes referred to as an infinitesimal model, was based on the idea that instead of concentrating entirely upon the effects of a few genes on a chosen human character, it would be beneficial to consider an infinitesimal number of genes and determine the aggregate effects of those genes on the character under investigation.

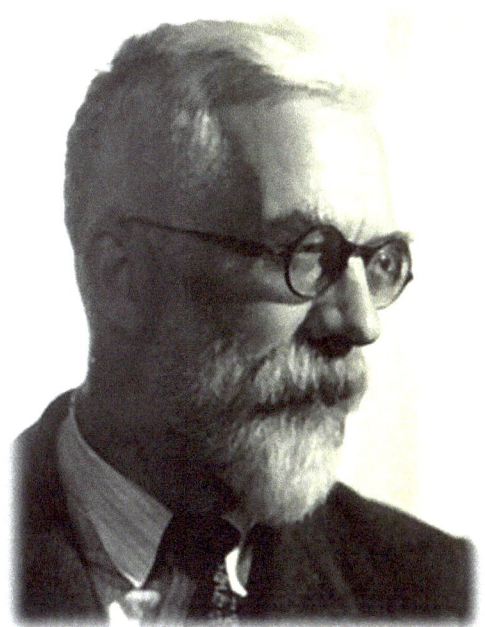

Figure 2.6
Sir Ronald Aylmer Fisher. Image courtesy of Special Collections, Barr Smith Library, The University of Adelaide.

Using this method, Fisher believed a better explanation could be provided of the action of genes, their individuality from each other and the smallest effect they could have in influencing a character. Fisher's model has been further developed to deal with the many complexities associated with understanding the quantitative genetics of human development.

It became a keystone upon which many future twin studies were based. Toward the end of his life in the late 1950s, Fisher lived in Adelaide, South Australia, visiting the Division of Mathematical Statistics in the Commonwealth Scientific Industrial Research Organisation (CSIRO). Working with Edmund A Cornish (Chief of Division, CSIRO) and J Henry Bennett, Professor of Genetics at the University of Adelaide, Fisher was able to influence many researchers. His 'Collected Papers' are still a source of inspiration to those involved with quantitative genetics. These papers were bound into five volumes and are stored in the archives in the University of Adelaide, Barr Smith Library (1995).

During his stay in Adelaide, many anecdotes were generated about Fisher, which added not only to his charisma but also to his impact as a teacher. Two well-remembered anecdotes, related to the authors of this book by Emeritus Professor Tasman Brown, illustrate the different memories people have of working with someone of the calibre of RA Fisher.

> 'I am sure Henry Bennett will have many memories to tell you. I remember he told me on one occasion that when Fisher was working on a problem on his desk electric-calculating machine, he would often pause at mid-stroke and stare out of the window for a long time and then when he had mentally solved the current problem, he would continue on the machine.'

> 'Sir Ronald was accustomed to dining in the University of Adelaide Staff Club and he would usually sit in a comfortable armchair and enjoy an after-lunch glass of milk. On one occasion Sir Ronald had dozed off but his peaceful slumber was rudely interrupted when one of the female dental patrons sitting at a nearby table accidentally swung her handbag, which sent Sir Ronald's glass flying. The esteemed statistician awoke with an audible start but was soon settled again by the profuse apologies from the shocked lady. Those in the dental school who were aware of this accident told the lady that by her carelessness she could have deprived the world of a revolutionary new statistical algorithm by waking Sir Ronald up too soon. The sad aftermath of the episode was the death of Sir Ronald soon after this event.'

References

Anon. (1680). *A true relation of a monstrous female-child, with two heads, four eyes, four ears, two noses, two mouths, and four arms, four legs, and all things else proportionably, fixed to one body.* London: Mallet.

Bondeson J (1993). The Isle-Brewers conjoined twins of 1680. *J R Soc Med* 86:106-109.

Bonnevie K (1924). Studies on papillary patterns of human fingers. *J Genet* 15:1-113.

Braund J, Sutton DG (2008). The case of Heinrich Wilhelm Poll (1877-1939): a German-Jewish geneticist, eugenicist, twin researcher, and victim of the Nazis. *J Hist Biol* 41:1-35.

Bryan EM (1983). *The nature and nurture of twins.* London: Baillère Tindall.

Burbridge D (2001). Francis Galton on twins, heredity and social class. *BJHS* 34:323-340.

Dahlberg G (1926). *Twin births and twins from a hereditary point of view.* Stockholm: Tidens.

Darwin C (1859). *On the origin of species.* London: John Murray.

Fisher RA (1936). Has Mendel's work been rediscovered? *Ann Sci* 1:115-137.

Fisher R, Bennett JH, Bennetto E, The Adelaide University Library (1995). 'Collected papers of RA Fisher, 1890-1962'. Adelaide: Adelaide University Library.

Galton F (1874). *English men of science: their nature and nurture.* London: Macmillan and Co.

Galton F (1875). The history of twins, as a criterion of the relative powers of nature and nurture. *Fraser's Mag* 12:566-576.

Galton F (1883). *Inquiries into human faculty and its development.* London: Macmillan and Co.

Gedda L (1961). *Twins in history and science.* Illinois: Charles C Thomas.

Gould SJ (1981). *The mismeasure of man.* New York: Norton.

Hunter J (1779). Account of the freemartin. *Phil Trans R Soc Lond* 69:279-293.

Huxley A (1932). *Brave new world.* London: Chatto & Windus.

Kompanje EJO (2004). The first successful separation of conjoined twins in 1689: some additions and corrections. *Twin Res* 7:537-541.

Lamarck JB (1809). *Philosophie Zoologique*. Paris: Chez Dentu.

Lauterbach CE (1925). Studies in twin resemblance. *Genetics* 10:525-568.

Locher J (1499). *Carmen Heroicum de Partu Monstrifero*. Ingolsladt: Johann Kachelofen.

Mayo O (2009). Early research on human genetics using the twin method: who really invented the method. *Twin Res Hum Genet* 12:237-245.

Merriman C (1924). The intellectual resemblance of twins. *Psychol Monogr* 33:1-57.

National Health and Medical Research Council, Australian Government (2007). *National Statement on Ethical Conduct in Human Research*, updated May 2015. http://www.nhmrc.gov.au/guidelines-publications/e72. Accessed 30 May 2015.

Newman HH (1928a). Studies of human twins: I. Methods of diagnosing monozygotic and dizygotic twins. *Biol Bull* 55:283-297.

Newman HH (1928b). Studies of human twins: II. Asymmetry reversal, of mirror imaging in identical twins. *Biol Bull* 55:298-315.

Newman HH (1934). Mental and physical traits of identical twins reared apart. *J Hered* 25:55-60.

Paré A (1575). *Des monstres et prodiges*. Translated into English with an introduction and notes by Pallister JL (1982). *On monsters and marvels*. Chicago: University of Chicago Press.

Pauls F (1969). Monoamniotic twin pregnancy: a review of the world literature and a report of two new cases. *Can Med Assoc J* 100:254-256.

Pearson K (1904). Mathematical contributions to the theory of evolution. XII. On a generalised theory of alternative inheritance, with special references to Mendel's laws. *Phil Trans R Soc Lond A* 203:53-86.

Poll H (1914). Über Zwillingsforschung als Hilfsmittel menschilcher Erbkunde. *Z Ethnol* 46:87-105.

Portin P (2014). The birth and development of the DNA theory of inheritance: sixty years since the discovery of the structure of DNA. *J Genet* 93:293-302.

Rende RD, Plomin R, Vandenberg SG (1990). Who discovered the twin method? *Behav Genet* 20:277-285.

Sand G. (1849). *La petite Fadette.* Paris: Calmann-Levy.

Siemens HW (1924). *Die Zwillingspathologie: ihre Bedeutung, ihre Methodik, ihre bisherigen Ergebnisse (The pathology of twins: significance, methodology, and results).* Berlin: Springer.

Siemens HW (1927). The diagnosis of identity in twins. *J Hered* 18:201-209.

Snow-Smith J (2004). *Leonardo da Vinci and printed ancient medical texts: history and influence.* Seattle: University of Washington.

Tallman GG (1928). A comparative study of identical and nonidentical twins with respect to intelligence resemblances. *27th Yrbk Nat Soc Studies Educ*:83-86.

Thorndike EL (1905). Measurements of twins. *Arch Phil Psych Sci Methods* 1:1-64.

Weinberg W (1901). Beiträgae zur Physiologie und Pathologie der Mehrlingsgeburten beim Menschen. *Arch Ges Physiol* 88:346-430.

Weinberg W (1910). Weitere Beiträge zur Theorie der Vererbung. *Arch Rass Ges Biol* 7:35-49.

Weitz W (1924). Studien an eineiigen Zwillingen. *Z Klin Med* 101:154.

Wilder T (1927). *The Bridge of San Luis Rey.* New York: Albert and Charles Boni.

Wilson PT, Jones HE (1932). Left-handedness in twins. *Genetics* 17:560-571.

Wingfield AH, Sandiford P (1928). Twins and orphans. *J Edu Psych* 19:410-423.

Chapter Three

PHASES OF RESEARCH INVOLVING TWIN STUDIES OF TEETH AND FACES

Three broad phases of research can be identified where twins have been studied to understand more about the contribution of genetic and environmental factors to human dental and facial variation. The number and types of studies have increased dramatically since the early 1900s.

STUDIES OF TWIN RESEMBLANCE: HEREDITARY AND ENVIRONMENTAL INFLUENCES

1920s-1940s

An initial phase of studies can be identified in the period from the 1920s to the early 1940s (see Table 3.1 at the end of this section for a summary of these studies). Several researchers around the world began studies of twins which highlighted resemblances of dental structures. Through being able to identify similarities in dental tissues they began to separate what could be thought of as genetically influenced (or hereditary) factors from environmentally influenced ones (Bachrach and Young, 1927; Goldberg, 1930; Korkhaus,1930; Newman 1923, 1928a,b, 1930; Newman et al.,1937). Indeed, publications involving Horatio H Newman commenced as early as 1913.

Henriette Bachrach and Matthew Young (1927) studied the resemblances of dental features in twin pairs who had been grouped into so-called identical pairs (development of more than one embryo from a fertilised egg) and non-identical pairs (development of embryos from separate fertilised eggs). The reason for forming these groupings conformed to the general belief that identical twin pairs shared the same inherited characteristics and that non-identical twin pairs shared only part of their inherited characteristics.

Using these two twin categories they set out to compare the degrees of influence that heredity and environment had upon chosen dental characteristics. These included tooth eruption times, dental caries in deciduous and permanent teeth, enamel hypoplasia, the state of dental occlusion and gingivitis. With the exception of total caries prevalence, data collected for all of the other features (particularly in subjects displaying different degrees of malocclusion) showed that correlations were higher in identical twin pairs than in non-identical twin pairs. This study and its choice of multiple dental features provided an important foundation for future studies involving dental morphology and disease in twins.

A paper written by Samuel Goldberg (1930) reported on dental arch size and shape in identical twins. His research considered resemblances of arch symmetry and asymmetry, as well as mirror imaging, in monozygotic twin pairs. Goldberg attempted to determine both the degree of arch variation and the severity of dental malocclusion. Using fifty sets of dental casts obtained from monozygotic twin pairs enrolled in Newman's University of Chicago studies, he concluded that arch symmetry and malocclusion were inherited. His assessment regarding malocclusion is interesting in that he makes the observation that teeth would be subject to 'intrinsic' pressures with hereditary influence on tooth position, as well as 'extrinsic' factors exerting an environmental effect. Such reasoning has orthodontic implications, in that attempts to prevent relapse of teeth to their original positions after treatment need to take account of the 'neutral zone' where the pressures exerted by the lips and cheeks are balanced by those of the tongue.

In all three phases involving research into dental variation, particularly research into malocclusion, researchers have often been orthodontists, or their research has been of value to orthodontic diagnosis and/or treatment. The fact that Goldberg used twin material from Newman's study emphasises the importance of the work conducted by Newman.

As early as 1913, Horatio H Newman was involved in understanding polyembryony (identical twin development) in armadillo species found in Texas and, in 1923, he conducted experiments on asymmetry in echinoderms (starfish). His work concerned identification of epigenetic factors related to polyembryony (that is, development of more than one embryo from a fertilised egg). The induced temperature variations upon the embryonic development of starfish eggs led him to consider the biological aspects of human twinning and higher order births.

Newman formulated a research programme on biological, statistical and psychological observations of identical and fraternal (non-identical) twins who were reared together (Newman, 1934). Later, it became possible to add data from identical twins reared apart. The dental component of this work was limited to observing dental irregularities and using this information to assist in determining twin zygosity. It was important because it brought together three distinct areas of study into a single research project concerning the rearing of twins (Newman et al., 1937). The fact that Newman's work began ten years before publication in 1937, and the fact that it was used by different researchers years later, shows the importance of data collections being shared in collaboration with other disciplines. Summarising this work, the three authors (Newman et al., 1937) noted that, despite generally higher correlations for identical twins, it was not possible to positively determine what influence genetic or environmental factors had upon the observed traits. They left the reader with the thought that 'what heredity can do environment can also do'.

Another paper by Gustav Korkhaus (1930) also considered questions relating to inherited dental characteristics. The difference between this paper and the others mentioned in this period is that Korkhaus used a different approach for his research. Instead of looking at subject data in a cross-sectional manner, he adopted a longitudinal approach to study facial and skull characteristics, tooth structure and size, colour of teeth and hypoplasia in twins. With regard to tooth size, Korkhaus felt that the observed variability in crown size of incisor teeth (particularly in lateral incisors) pointed to definite genetic causation. He also noted that 'only a large number of cases will justify distinct conclusions ... whereon to enlarge continuously will be our next task'.

Because Korkhaus was open-minded about his observations, he accepted criticism over some of his conclusions. For example, he admitted that his opinion that the diastema (a space between front teeth) was an inherited characteristic was open to question (Figure 3.1).

Earlier work had raised the issue of what constituted a diastema (Siemens and Hunold, 1924), and Korkhaus realised that without clear guidelines to define the extent of spacing between teeth, it was impossible to accurately record the feature.

Phases of research involving twin studies of teeth and faces

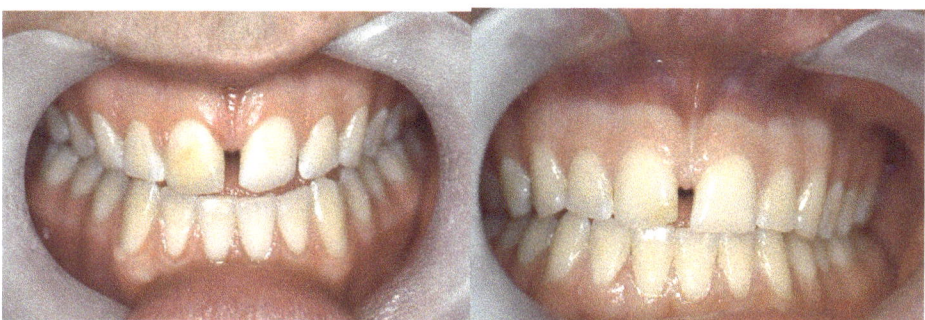

Figure 3.1
Diastema in a pair of monozygotic twin boys.

Today, researchers measure dental variables with high degrees of accuracy using either direct methods — for example, high-precision callipers — or indirectly, using 2D or 3D digital imaging systems.

In the late 1940s, Anders Lundström, Professor of Orthodontics at the Karolinska Institutet in Stockholm, Sweden, published two landmark papers on dental occlusion and malocclusion in twins (Figure 3.2).

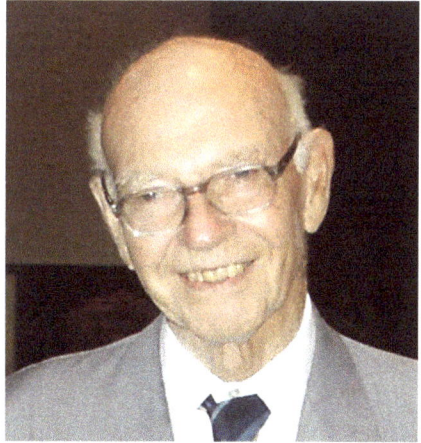

Figure 3.2
Professor Anders Lundström, Karolinska Institutet, Stockholm.
Photograph courtesy of Professor Jan Huggare, Department of Dental Medicine, Karolinska Institute, Huddinge, Sweden. We acknowledge with thanks Fredric Lundström for allowing this photograph of his father to be published in this book.

In the late 1940s, Anders Lundström (1948, 1949) considered tooth size in twins and the causal background of various types of malocclusion. In his study of malocclusion, he reasoned that environmental factors included two categories: internal and external.

The concept of an internal component is compatible with the physiological notion of the 'milieu intérieur', whereby homeostatic mechanisms attempt to maintain a constant environment within the individual. This idea of two environmental components acting within and outside the body was considered earlier by Gunnar Dahlberg (1948). Lundström was influenced by Dahlberg's work, and felt that variation in tooth position was associated with the internal factor. He also considered that this variation occurred at random. To this end he structured his study to determine what percentage of the observed variation could be attributed to random factors, and what could not. Through identification of the random element he was able to construct clearly distinguished categories between what he felt were external, internal and hereditary causation factors. This approach enabled Lundström to more accurately define the environmental component affecting variation associated with malocclusion.

Table 3.1

Key studies of the teeth and faces of twins 1920s-1940s

Researchers	Country	Date	Key publications
Siemens HW	Germany	1927	*The diagnosis of identity in twins*
Bachrach FH, Young M	England	1927	*A comparison of the degree of resemblance in dental characters shown in pairs of twins of identical and fraternal types*
Goldberg S	USA	1929	*Biometrics of identical twins from the dental viewpoint*
Goldberg S	USA	1930	*The dental arches of identical twins*
Korkhaus G	Germany	1930	*Anthropologic and odontologic studies of twins*
Newman HH et al.	USA	1937	*Twins: a study of heredity and environment*
Lundström A	Sweden	1948	*Tooth size and occlusion in twins*
Lundström A	Sweden	1949	*An investigation of 202 pairs of twins regarding fundamental factors in the aetiology of malocclusion*

Phases of research involving twin studies of teeth and faces

UNDERSTANDING GENETIC CONTROL OVER DENTAL VARIATION

1950s-1980s

The second phase of dental research involving twins can be considered to have spanned the years from the 1950s to the 1980s (see Table 3.2 at the end of this section for a summary of this research). The key researchers in this phase continued with attempts to define the extent of genetic control over dental variation using more sophisticated methods. One focus was to clarify the aetiology of dental occlusion and malocclusion. Leading researchers during this period were Richard Osborne and Sidney Horowitz in the USA (Horowitz et al., 1958a,b; Osborne et al., 1958), Anders Lundström in Sweden (Lundström, 1954), and Stanley Garn at the Fels Research Institute in Ohio, USA (Garn et al., 1965).

This period also saw the extended use of odontometrics. Osborne and his colleagues concentrated their research on the hereditary factors influencing variation in anterior tooth size and occlusion in monozygotic (MZ) and dizygotic (DZ) twins (Figure 3.3).

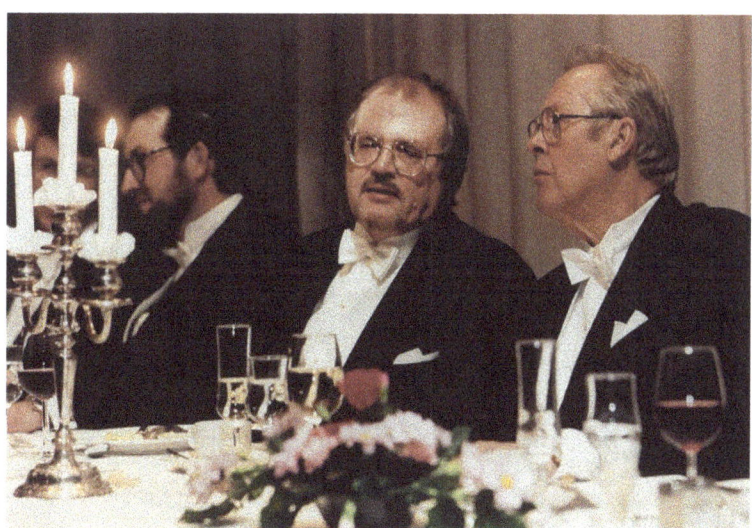

Figure 3.3
Professor Lassi Alvesalo (centre) pictured with Professor Richard H Osborne (far right) in Oulu (May 1996). Photograph courtesy Professor Tuomo Heikkinen (far left), Institute of Dentistry, University of Oulu, Finland.

Using twin pairs enrolled in the Collaborative Perinatal Study of the National Institute of Neurological Disorders and Stroke, they recorded information on ethnicity, geographic background and religion. Zygosity was determined through blood group factors and through observed similarities in physical structures. Osborne and his colleagues also obtained dental radiographs and impressions of the mouths of their subjects and poured casts in dental stone. These casts enabled measurements of the teeth to be made, which provided odontometric data for analysis. They concluded that there was a strong genetic influence on variability of mesiodistal crown dimensions of permanent anterior teeth. Osborne, like many other dental anthropologists, believed in sharing information with colleagues around the world. He attended numerous dental morphological symposia and organised access for others to the databases used in his research. The ability to access twin databases throughout the world is becoming more and more important in building adequate sample sizes to address research questions.

Without doubt, Stanley Garn was one of the key figures in physical anthropology in the twentieth century (Figure 3.4). He was a prolific author of many papers, some of which relied on data obtained from twins in relation to body composition, skeletal development and dental development. An important event in Garn's life occurred when he joined the Department of Physical Growth and Genetics at the Fels Research

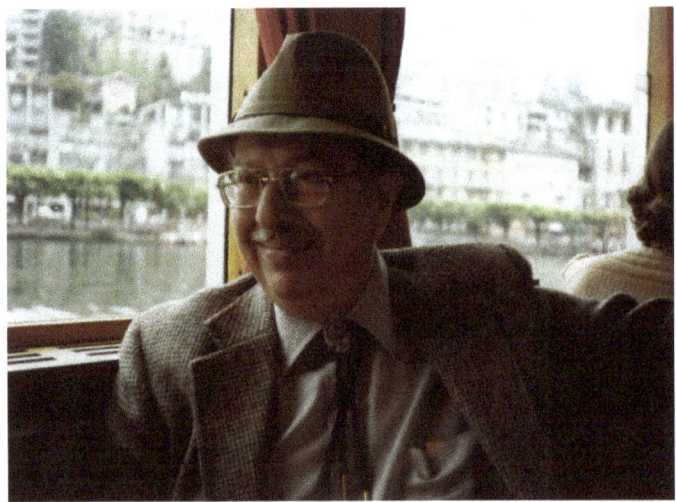

Figure 3.4
Stanley M Garn (1922-2007).
Photograph courtesy of B Holly Smith, University of Michigan.

Phases of research involving twin studies of teeth and faces

Institute in Yellow Springs, Ohio, USA. Becoming its chairman in 1952, Garn became responsible for enlarging the physical anthropology component within the Fels database, and he was also instrumental in its development into the most extensive, and longest running, continuous longitudinal growth study in the world. Many of his publications were derived from this extensive database. The sixteen years he spent at Fels enabled him to broaden his interests in research into human growth, population epidemiology and family-related genetic studies. His work on the genetics of dental development including siblings and twins became a blueprint for future studies (Garn, 1977).

Another early and extensive longitudinal twin study into growth and dental development of monozygotic and dizygotic twins was undertaken in 1959 by Coenraad Moorrees at the Forsyth Dental Centre in Boston, USA (Figure 3.5). Moorrees, working with Anna-Maria Grøn and Laure Lebret, developed a database to which they added orthodontic and anthropometric measurements for the next twenty years. Over 400 twin pairs were involved, aged between 6 to 16 years. Records of parents and non-twin siblings were also included in the database. Unfortunately, relatively few publications resulted from this ambitious study, apparently due to funding inadequacies (Peck and Will, 2004).

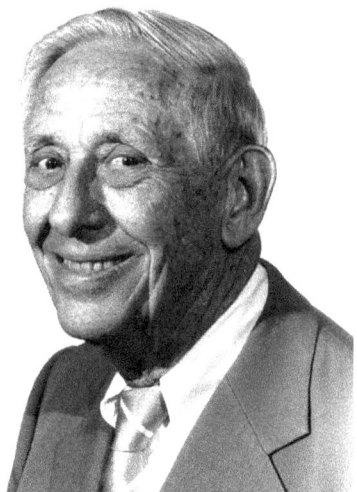

Figure 3.5
Coenraad F. A. Moorrees (1916-2003).
Reprinted from the American Journal of Orthodontics and Dentofacial Orthopedics. Copyright 2004 with permission from Elsevier.

Although the statistical analyses that were available during this period were limited to simple variance ratios and correlations, the researchers of this time provided many of the ground rules for future research. In the latter half of this era, more sophisticated analyses of twin data became possible, with greater access to increasing computer power. There was also a growing awareness that the various assumptions of the twin model needed to be tested rigorously before calculating estimates of genetic variance. In the 1970s, Joe Christian and colleagues undertook research to estimate genetic variance for various features in twins and also to construct a basic methodology for twin analysis (Christian et al., 1974; Christian, 1979). Consideration was also given to the assertion that monozygotic co-twins were likely to share more similar environments postnatally than dizygotic co-twins. This led to the testing of the 'equal environments assumption' (that both monozygotic and dizygotic co-twins shared similar environments), which had been a centrepiece of the classical twin study paradigm. This was particularly relevant when considering the development of psychological traits in twins and how those traits could be affected in different environments.

The development of a twin model which considered genetic and environmental factors acting upon monozygotic and dizygotic twin pairs who had been reared apart from birth provided a way of overcoming the problem of similar environments affecting features in co-twins. However, the 'twins reared apart' model has assumptions of its own, most of which are related to the different twin environments and how these environments may affect measured characteristics in individual co-twins (Bouchard, 2006).

Some of the key researchers during this time were Robert Biggerstaff in Kentucky (Biggerstaff, 1970, 1975), Rose Potter in Indianapolis (Potter et al., 1976), Robert Corruccini in Illinois (Corruccini and Potter, 1980), Minuro Nakata in Japan (Nakata et al., 1973, 1974; Nakata, 1985), Yuji Mizoguchi in Japan (1977), and Winfried Harzer in Germany (Harzer, 1987). In addition to studies estimating genetic contributions to observed variation of teeth, there was increasing interest in exploring the nature and causes of asymmetry within the dentition using data obtained from twins (Potter and Nance, 1976).

Not only were the traditional measures of dental crown size used in these analyses, but variations in cusp expression and crown components were also explored (Staley and Greene, 1974; Corruccini and Potter, 1981). Another researcher, Charles Boklage, placed the investigation of dental asymmetry in twins into a broader biological context and proposed that craniofacial development in twins differed from that in singletons, and that this difference was related in some way to the biological basis of the twinning process (Boklage, 1987). This work provides an important reminder of the need to test whether data derived from twins can be extrapolated to the general population.

It was not until the 1990s that statistical approaches based upon path analysis and model-fitting could be applied. These approaches enabled estimations of the different contributions of genetic and environmental factors to phenotypic variation to be made and the fit of different models to be tested statistically.

Table 3.2
Key studies of the teeth and faces of twins 1950s-1980s

Researchers	Country	Date	Key publications
Lundström A	Sweden	1954	*The importance of genetic and non-genetic factors in the facial skeleton studied in 100 pairs of twins*
Horowitz SL et al.	USA	1958a	*Caries experience in twins*
Horowitz SL et al.	USA	1958b	*Hereditary factors in tooth dimensions, a study of the anterior teeth of twins*
Osborne RH DeGeorge FV	USA	1959	*Genetic basis of morphological variation: an evaluation and application of the twin study method*
Kraus BS et al.	USA	1959	*Heredity and the craniofacial complex*
Hunter WS	USA	1959	*The inheritance of mesiodistal tooth diameter in twins*
Horowitz SL et al.	USA	1960	*A cephalometric study of craniofacial variation in adult twins*
Osborne RH	USA	1961	*Applications of twin studies to dental research*
Horowitz SL	USA	1963	*Clinical aspects of genetic research in dentistry*
Lundström A	Sweden	1963	*Tooth morphology as a basis for distinguishing monozygotic and dizygotic twins*
Garn S et al.	USA	1965	*Genetic, nutritional, and maturational correlates of dental development*
Hunter WS	USA	1965	*A study of the inheritance of craniofacial characteristics as seen in lateral cephalograms of 72 like-sexed twins*
Mulick JF	USA	1965	*An investigation of craniofacial asymmetry using the serial twin-study method*
Keene HJ	USA	1968	*Discordant dental development in twins*

Twin Studies

Researchers	Country	Date	Key publications
Shapiro BL	USA	1969	*A twin study of palatal dimensions partitioning genetic and environmental contributions to variability*
Biggerstaff RH	USA	1970	*Morphological variations for the permanent mandibular first molars in human monozygotic and dizygotic twins*
Keene HJ	USA	1971	*Birth weight and congenital absence of teeth in twins*
Staley RN, Green LJ	USA	1971	*Bilateral asymmetry in tooth cusp occurrence in human monozygotic twins, dizygotic twins, and nontwins*
Nakata M et al.	Japan, USA	1974	*Genetic determinants of cranio-facial morphology: a twin study*
Biggerstaff RH	USA	1975	*Cusp size, sexual dimorphism, and heritability of cusp size in twins*
Potter R, Nance W	USA	1976	*A twin study of dental dimension. I. Discordance, asymmetry, and mirror imagery*
Potter RH et al.	USA	1976	*A twin study of dental dimension. II. Independent genetic determinants*
Rebich T, Markovic M	USA, Yugoslavia	1976	*Inheritance of tooth dimension: a quantitative genetic twin study*
Garn SM	USA	1977	*Genetics of dental development*
Mizoguchi Y	Japan	1977	*Genetic variability of permanent tooth crowns as ascertained from twin data*
Kent RL et al.	USA	1978	*Associations in emergence age among permanent teeth*
Corruccini RS, Potter RHY	USA	1980	*Genetic analysis of occlusal variation in twins*
Markovic M	Yugoslavia	1982	*Hypodontia in twins*
Sognnaes RF et al.	USA	1982	*Computer comparison of bitemark patterns in identical twins*
Boklage CE	USA	1984	*Differences in protocols of craniofacial development related to twinship and zygosity*
Hauspie RC et al.	Belgium	1985	*Testing for the presence of genetic variance in factors of face measurements of Belgian twins*
Boraas JC et al.	USA	1988	*A genetic contribution to dental caries, occlusion, and morphology as demonstrated by twins reared apart*
Nyström M, Ranta R	Finland	1988	*Dental age and asymmetry in the formation of mandibular teeth in twins concordant or discordant for oral clefts*
Townsend GC et al.	Australia	1988	*Genetic and environmental determinants of dental occlusal variation in South Australian twins*

Phases of research involving twin studies of teeth and faces

DEVELOPMENT OF MORE SOPHISTICATED METHODS: PATH ANALYSIS, MODEL-FITTING AND GENETIC EXPRESSION

1990s to the present

A third phase of research relating to dental and facial development in twins extends from the 1990s to the present (see Table 3.3 at the end of this section for a summary of this research). This period has seen increasing application of statistical approaches based on path analysis and model-fitting, whereby models incorporating different contributions of genetic and environmental factors to phenotypic variation can be applied to data and tested statistically for their goodness of fit. Initially, the computer program LISREL was applied to dental data, but then an improved version of LISREL, referred to as Mx, was applied (Neale, 1995).

A study of dental and facial morphology in Australian twins commenced in Adelaide in 1983 and, following discussions at the 7th International Symposium on Dental Morphology in Paris in 1986, a collaborative approach to data analysis was adopted between Rob Corruccini and Grant Townsend (Townsend et al., 1988; Corruccini et al., 1990). As the number of twins enrolled in the Australian study increased, a further collaboration was developed with Professor Louise Brearley Messer in Melbourne, Australia, with Professor Brearley Messer focusing particularly on the analysis of facial morphology (Tangchaitrong et al., 2000).

With the encouragement and support of Nick Martin, an Australian and a key international figure in twin research, model-fitting methods began to be applied to dental data in the 1990s (Townsend and Martin, 1992; Dempsey et al., 1995). With ever-increasing computer power and technology it has become possible to carry out more sophisticated analyses. One researcher in Adelaide involved in this process is Toby Hughes, who has applied structural equation modelling to data from twins. An important benefit provided by Hughes's work has been clarification of the sources of covariation between correlated variables derived from longitudinal data (Hughes et al., 2000; Townsend et al., 2003; Hughes et al., 2007).

A recent innovative method of understanding the effect of genes upon developing dental features is the use of GWAS (Genome-Wide Association Studies). This method involves the use of large twin and family cohort collections to identify genetic variants or loci responsible for the dental feature under review. Current dental research using GWAS has involved the identification of genes at designated loci which are associated with primary and permanent tooth emergence (Pillas et al., 2010; Geller et al., 2011). The ability to identify gene expression on developing phenotypes is not limited to tooth emergence, but is proving to be valuable in research into other dental and body organ development. It has also been of value in determining loci implicated in the development of ovarian, breast and colorectal cancer.

Genetic research has moved beyond analysing phenotypic variability into the realm of exploring the aetiology of disease. The search for genetic markers using classical twin study methods has made inroads into understanding the biological mechanisms of disease. One example of this type of research is a study which compared the DNA methylation patterns of discordant monozygotic twins. DNA methylation is a controlling factor in gene expression (Bell and Spector, 2011). Methylation changes, or differences in epigenetic profiles, were noted in twins who were discordant for systemic lupus erythematosus (van Dongen et al., 2012).

Genetically inspired research into the aetiology of dental development is becoming more involved with understanding the communication pathways between cells and tissues during cellular differentiation. Multifactorial interactions of genetic, epigenetic and environmental influences are thought to contribute to various dental anomalies, including variations in tooth size, shape, number and structure (Brook, 2009; Brook et al., 2014). Already, over 300 genes have been associated with dental development (Thesleff 2006; Créton et al., 2013).

A large-scale study of oral health in twins is currently being undertaken by Walter Bretz at New York University, together with other colleagues in the USA. Bretz has collected data from over 1000 pairs of twins living in disadvantaged areas of Montes Claros in Brazil. Because there is inadequate fluoridation of the water supply and also poor access to dental care, the children in the study are at risk of developing dental caries. The study aims to determine the importance of genetic and environmental influences on the development of dental caries, and involves comparisons between monozygotic and dizygotic twin pairs, as well as comparisons between monozygotic co-twins where one has evidence of dental caries and the other does not (Bretz et al., 2006; Corby et al., 2007).

Phases of research involving twin studies of teeth and faces

Table 3.3
Key studies of the teeth and faces of twins 1990s to the present

Researchers	Country	Date	Key publications
Coruccini RS et al.	USA, Australia	1990	*Genetic and environmental determinants of dental occlusal variation in twins of different nationalities*
Markovic MD	Yugoslavia	1992	*At the crossroads of oral facial genetics*
Townsend GC Martin NG	Australia	1992	*Fitting genetic models to Carabelli trait data in South Australian twins*
Dempsey PJ et al.	Australia	1995	*Genetic covariance structure of incisor crown size in twins*
Carels C, Vlietinck R	Belgium	1999	*Role of inheritability of tooth form, tooth malformation and tooth position*
Tangchaitrong K et al.	Australia	2000	*Fourier analysis of facial profiles of young twins*
Kabban M et al.	UK	2001	*Tooth size and morphology in twins*
Townsend G et al.	Australia	2003	*Molar intercuspal dimensions: genetic input to phenotypic variation*
Bretz WA et al.	USA	2005a	*Dental caries and microbial acid production in twins*
Bretz WA et al.	USA	2005b	*Longitudinal analysis of heritability for dental caries traits*
Corby PM et al.	USA	2005	*Mutans streptococci in preschool twins*
Bretz WA et al.	USA	2006	*Heritability estimates for dental caries and sucrose sweetness preference*
Hughes TE et al.	Australia	2007	*Strong genetic control of emergence of human primary incisors*
Corby PM et al.	USA	2007	*Heritability of oral microbial species in caries-active and caries-free twins*
Su C-Y et al.	USA	2008	*Inheritance of occlusal topography: a twin study*
Boklage CE	USA	2010	*How new humans are made*
Bockmann MR et al.	Australia	2011	*Timing of colonization of caries-producing bacteria: an approach based on studying monozygotic twins*
Hughes T et al.	Australia, UK	2012	*Genetic, epigenetic, and environmental influences on dentofacial structures and oral health: ongoing studies of Australian twins and their families*
Ribeiro DC et al.	Australia, UK	2013	*Intrauterine hormone effects on tooth dimensions*
Hughes T et al.	Australia, UK	2014	*The teeth and faces of twins: providing insights into dentofacial development and oral health for practising oral health professionals*

Twin Studies

STUDIES OF TWINS: THE ADELAIDE DENTAL SCHOOL

The genesis of the studies of twins in the Adelaide Dental School can be traced back to Grant Townsend's experiences as a PhD student under the supervision of Professor Tasman Brown. Having completed his PhD on variation in tooth size within the Aboriginal people from Yuendumu in Central Australia, and after publishing some papers presenting these findings, Townsend began thinking about commencing another study to provide further insights into the roles of genetic and environmental influences on variation in human tooth size.

His PhD had used a special familial relationship that existed amongst the Yuendumu Aboriginal people to explore the roles of genetic and environmental factors on tooth size variation. These people practised a custom of polygyny, where a male could have more than one wife. There were also very detailed genealogical records available of the family groupings that had been collected by Murray Barrett (Fleming et al., 1971). Therefore, it was possible to look at the similarities in tooth size and morphology in full-siblings and also half-siblings who had the same father but different mothers. Data of this type are very rare and the relationships enabled the researchers to calculate not only the heritability estimates — that is, how much of the variation in features could be explained by genetic influences — but also how much of the variation could be attributed to so-called common environmental influences or maternal effects. These analyses highlighted a strong genetic influence on tooth size variation, but also showed for the first time that there was a significant maternal effect, presumably due to prenatal, and possibly perinatal, influences during dental development.

Given that the sample sizes were relatively small in the Yuendumu sample, Townsend was keen to explore another sample and to build up larger numbers of subjects. This is particularly important when attempting to calculate accurate estimates of heritability. Drawing on his experiences studying genetics and human variation with Professor Henry Bennett during his Honours year, and drawing also on discussions with Nick Martin who tutored in the course, Townsend began thinking about a study of tooth size and shape in twins. He was aware of the value of twin studies that compared monozygotic pairs with dizygotic pairs, and he was also aware of new, more sophisticated statistical techniques that were beginning to be used to analyse data derived from twins.

Phases of research involving twin studies of teeth and faces

Townsend's experiences of the Yuendumu Growth Study with Tasman Brown and Murray Barrett (Brown et al., 2011) reinforced his appreciation of the value of longitudinal human growth studies. He also realised that if any growth studies were to be performed in Australia that focused on dental features, the people most likely to be able to perform the research would be dental academics working in a university environment. This is because of the huge commitment of time and effort needed to plan and run long-term growth studies, with the need for some stability in terms of ongoing staffing and resources, including storage of the records that are collected.

Townsend had seen how the records and information collected during the years of the Yuendumu Growth Study had served as a focus for postgraduate students and for national and international visitors who wanted to study the material. Although the dental casts of Indigenous Australians had been collected in the 1950s, 1960s and early 1970s, they were still being regularly accessed as new research questions arose — and they still are! Townsend could see that much of the Adelaide School of Dentistry's international reputation for research had been built around publications and presentations based on the unique collection of growth records of the Yuendumu Aboriginal people. He was keen to further build this reputation by gathering additional records, such as dental casts of twins, to complement the Yuendumu study.

Grant Townsend, Tasman Brown and Lindsay Richards, together with Sandy Pinkerton, began developing plans in the early 1980s for a study of twins living in South Australia. They were helped greatly by advice from Nick Martin. It was essential to gain some funding to support the study and it was felt that a longitudinal study might be too ambitious as an initial project. Tasman Brown had a particular interest in facial development and morphology, so the group decided to focus on the teeth and faces of twins. They also felt that teenage twins would be more comfortable with having impressions made of their teeth and giving blood samples for the determination of zygosities than younger twins would be. The plan was to enrol around 300 pairs of teenage twins in the study, mainly in the age range of 12 to 15 years, as these twins would have all of their permanent teeth present except for the third molars. With the assistance of the NHMRC (National Health and Medical Research Council) Twin Registry located in Melbourne, and with financial support from the NHMRC, the examination of twins commenced in April 1983 and was completed in 1993. While this study, now referred to as Cohort 1, was to be a cross-sectional study, it was always hoped that the research would proceed well, and that a subsequent longitudinal study might be possible at some stage in the future. A fuller description of the Cohort 1 study is provided in Chapter Four.

In 1995, a longitudinal growth study of twins around 4 to 6 years of age was commenced, with a view to examining the twins on at least two more occasions. It was planned to examine approximately 300 pairs of twins when all the primary teeth were present, then again when there were both primary and permanent teeth (the mixed dentition stage around 9 to 11 years of age) and then again when all the permanent teeth were present apart from third molars (around 12 to 14 years of age). This group of twins, together with their brothers and sisters, is now referred to as Cohort 2. With continuing support from the NHMRC, as well as Colgate and the ADRF (Australian Dental Research Foundation), the examinations of twins in Cohort 2 continued throughout the 1990s, to be completed in 2006. Many of the twins being examined were seen in the Dental Therapy School Melbourne, with colleague Professor Louise Brearley Messer. More details about the Cohort 2 study are provided in Chapter Five.

In 2003, following discussions with Professor Kim Seow in Brisbane, Queensland, and Professor Theo Gotjamanos in Perth, Western Australia, it was decided to broaden the focus of the twin studies by including consideration of oral health. Toby Hughes and Michelle Bockmann, who were now part of the Craniofacial Biology Research Group, took leading roles in this new phase, referred to as Cohort 3. A novel aspect of this study was to ask the parents of the twins to record when primary teeth appeared in the mouth, rather than requiring all of the twins to come to the Dental School for clinical examinations. Advances in technology also enabled the parents to obtain samples of dental plaque from the teeth, and to use buccal swabs to obtain samples of DNA for zygosity determination. This study is ongoing and is described in Chapter Six.

Whilst twin research in the Adelaide School of Dentistry is ongoing, the thought patterns and events described above are likely to be re-enacted worldwide amongst researchers attempting to explain the causes of variation in human dental and facial development. Two aspects that are likely to be central to the future of these types of twin studies are increasing collaboration between researchers internationally and the ability of those researchers to gain access to large databases of twins and their families while ensuring that all ethical issues are addressed.

Given our similar research interests, we have entered into an exciting new phase of collaboration with Walter Bretz and his colleagues in the USA. The twins involved in our respective studies represent the two largest samples currently available worldwide for exploring the roles of genetic and environmental influences on oral health and disease. While combining resources promises to enable some key questions to be addressed, we are very conscious of the need to ensure that genomic data are managed with the highest levels of ethical behaviour. It is very important that we adopt the most appropriate approaches to the ethical management of genomic data obtained from our twins and their families. A paper by Jean McEwen and colleagues has recently reviewed the challenges and possible future directions in dealing with this issue in such changing times (McEwen et al., 2013).

References

Bachrach FH, Young M (1927). A comparison of the degree of resemblance in dental characters shown in pairs of twins of identical and fraternal types. *Brit Dent J* XLVIII:1293-1304.

Bell JT, Spector TD (2011). A twin approach to unraveling epigenetics. *Trends Genet* 27:116-125.

Biggerstaff RH (1970). Morphological variations for the permanent mandibular first molars in human monozygotic and dizygotic twins. *Arch Oral Biol* 15:721-730.

Biggerstaff RH (1975). Cusp size, sexual dimorphism, and heritability of cusp size in twins. *Am J Phys Anthropol* 42:127-140.

Bockmann MR, Harris AV, Bennett CN, Odeh R, Hughes TE, Townsend GC (2011). Timing of colonization of caries-producing bacteria: an approach based on studying monozygotic twin pairs. *Int J Dent* Article ID 571573. doi:10.1155/2011/571573. Accessed 19 May 2015.

Boklage CE (1984). Differences in protocols of craniofacial development related to twinship and zygosity. *J Craniofac Genet Dev Biol* 4:151-169.

Boklage CE (1987). Developmental differences between singletons and twins in distributions of dental diameter asymmetries. *Am J Phys Anthropol* 74:319-331.

Boklage CE (2010). *How new humans are made*. Singapore: World Scientific Publishing Co. Pte Ltd.

Boraas JC, Messer LB, Till MJ (1988). A genetic contribution to dental caries, occlusion, and morphology as demonstrated by twins reared apart. *J Dent Res* 67:1150-1155.

Bouchard TJ Jr (2006). Identical twins reared apart. In: *eLS*. Chichester: John Wiley & Sons Ltd. http://www.els.net. doi:10.1038/npg.els.0005156. Accessed 19 May 2015.

Bretz WA, Corby PM, Hart TC, Costa S, Coelho MQ, Weyant RJ, et al. (2005a). Dental caries and microbial acid production in twins. *Caries Res* 39:168-172.

Bretz WA, Corby PM, Schork NJ, Robinson MT, Coelho M, Costa S, et al. (2005b). Longitudinal analysis of heritability for dental caries traits. *J Dent Res* 84:1047-1051.

Bretz WA, Corby PMA, Melo MR, Coelho MQ, Costa SM, Robinson M, et al. (2006). Heritability estimates for dental caries and sucrose sweetness preference. *Arch Oral Biol* 51:1156-1160.

Brook AH (2009). Multilevel complex interactions between genetic, epigenetic and environmental factors in the aetiology of anomalies of dental development. *Arch Oral Biol* 54(1 Suppl):S3-S17.

Brook AH, Jernvall J, Smith RN, Hughes TE, Townsend GC (2014). The dentition: the outcomes of morphogenesis leading to variations of tooth number, size and shape. *Aust Dent J* 59 (1 Suppl):131-142.

Brown T, Townsend GC, Pinkerton SK, Rogers JR (2011). *Yuendumu: legacy of a longitudinal growth study in Central Australia.* Adelaide: University of Adelaide Press.

Carels C, Vlietinck R (1999). Role of inheritability of tooth form, tooth malformation and tooth position. *Ned Tijdschr Tandheelkd* 106: 298-301.

Christian JC (1979). Testing twin means and estimating genetic variance: basic methodology for the analysis of quantitative twin data. *Acta Genet Med Gemellol* 28:35-40.

Christian JC, Kang KW, Norton JA Jr (1974). Choice of an estimate of genetic variance from twin data. *Am J Hum Genet* 26:154-161.

Corby PM, Bretz WA, Hart TC, Filho MM, Oliveira B, Vanyukov M (2005). Mutans streptococci in preschool twins. *Arch Oral Biol* 50:347-351.

Corby PM, Bretz WA, Hart TC, Schork NJ, Wessel J, Lyons-Weiler J, et al. (2007). Heritability of oral microbial species in caries-active and caries-free twins. *Twin Res Hum Genet* 10:821-828.

Corruccini RS, Potter RHY (1980). Genetic analysis of occlusal variation in twins. *Am J Orthod* 78:140-154.

Corruccini RS, Potter RHY (1981). Developmental correlates of crown component asymmetry and occlusal discrepancy. *Am J Phys Anthropol* 55:21-31.

Corruccini RS, Townsend GC, Richards LC, Brown T (1990). Genetic and environmental determinants of dental occlusal variation in twins of different nationalities. *Hum Biol* 62:353-367.

Créton M, van den Boogaard MJ, Maal T, Verhamme L, Fennis W, Carels C, et al. (2013). Three-dimensional analysis of tooth dimensions in the *MSX1*-missense mutation. *Clin Oral Invest* 17:1437-1445.

Dahlberg G (1948). Environment, inheritance and random variation with special reference to investigations on twins. *Acta Genet Stat Med* 1:104-114.

Dempsey PJ, Townsend GC, Martin NG, Neale MC (1995). Genetic covariance structure of incisor crown size in twins. *J Dent Res* 74:1389-1398.

Fleming DA, Barrett MJ, Fleming TJ (1971). Family records of an Australian community. *Abor Stud News* 3:15.

Garn SM (1977). Genetics of dental development. In: *The Biology of Occlusal Development*. McNamara JA, editor. Ann Arbor: Center for Human Growth and Development. pp. 61-88.

Garn SM, Lewis AB, Kerewsky RS (1965). Genetic, nutritional, and maturational correlates of dental development. *J Dent Res* 44:228-242.

Geller F, Feenstra B, Zhang H, Shaffer JR, Hansen T, Esserlind A-L, et al. (2011). Genome-wide association study identifies four loci associated with eruption of permanent teeth. *PLoS Genet* 2011;7: e1002275. doi:10.1371/journal.pgen.1002275. Accessed 19 May 2015.

Goldberg S (1929). Biometrics of identical twins from the dental viewpoint. *J Dent Res* 9:363-409.

Goldberg S (1930). The dental arches of identical twins. *Dent Cosmos* 72:869-881.

Gould SJ (1981). *The mismeasure of man.* New York: WW Norton & Co.

Harzer W (1987). A hypothetical model of genetic control of tooth-crown growth in man. *Arch Oral Biol* 32:159-162.

Hauspie RC, Susanne C, Defrise-Gussenhoaven E (1985). Testing for the presence of genetic variance in factors of face measurements of Belgian twins. *Ann Hum Biol* 12:429-440.

Horowitz SL (1963). Clinical aspects of genetic research in dentistry. *J Dent Res* 42:1330-1343.

Horowitz SL, Osborne RH, DeGeorge FV (1958a). Caries experience in twins. *Science* 128:300-301.

Horowitz SL, Osborne RH, DeGeorge FV (1958b). Hereditary factors in tooth dimensions, a study of the anterior teeth of twins. *Angle Orthod* 28:87-93.

Horowitz SL, Osborne RH, DeGeorge FV (1960). A cephalometric study of craniofacial variation in adult twins. *Angle Orthod* 30:1-5.

Hughes T, Dempsey P, Richards L, Townsend G (2000). Genetic analysis of deciduous tooth size in Australian twins. *Arch Oral Biol* 11:997-1004.

Hughes T, Bockmann M, Mihailidis S, Bennett C, Harris A, Seow WK, et al. (2012). Genetic, epigenetic, and environmental influences on dentofacial structures and oral health: ongoing studies of Australian twins and their families. *Twin Res Hum Genet* 16:43-51.

Hughes TE, Bockmann MR, Seow K, Gotjamanos T, Gully N, Richards LC, et al. (2007). Strong genetic control of emergence of human primary incisors. *J Dent Res* 86:1160-1165.

Hughes TE, Townsend GC, Pinkerton SK, Bockmann MR, Seow WK, Brook AH, et al. (2014). The teeth and faces of twins: providing insights into dentofacial development and oral health for practising oral health professionals. *Aust Dent J* 59 (1 Suppl):101-116.

Hunter WS (1959). *The inheritance of mesiodistal tooth diameter in twins.* Thesis, University of Michigan, Ann Arbor.

Hunter WS (1965). A study of the inheritance of craniofacial characteristics as seen in lateral cephalograms of 72 like-sexed twins. *Rep Congr Eur Orthod Soc* 41:59-70.

Kabban M, Fearne J, Jovanovski V, Zou L (2001). Tooth size and morphology in twins. *Int J Paediatr Dent* 11:333-339.

Keene HJ (1968). Discordant dental development in twins. *J Dent Res* 47:175.

Keene HJ (1971). Birth weight and congenital absence of teeth in twins. *Acta Genet Med Gemellol* 20:23-42.

Kent RL Jr, Reed RB, Moorrees CFA (1978). Associations in emergence age among permanent teeth. *Am J Phys Anthropol* 48:131-142.

Korkhaus G (1930). Anthropologic and odontologic studies of twins. *Int J Orthod Oral Surg Rad* 16:640-647.

Kraus BS, Wise WJ, Frei RH (1959). Heredity and the craniofacial complex. *Am J Orthodont* 45:172-217.

Lundström A (1948). *Tooth size and occlusion in twins*. Basel: Karger.

Lundström A (1949). An investigation of 202 pairs of twins regarding fundamental factors in the aetiology of malocclusion. *Dent Rec* LXIX:251-264.

Lundström A (1954). The importance of genetic and non-genetic factors in the facial skeleton studied in 100 pairs of twins. *Eur Orthod Soc Rep Cong* 30:92-107.

Lundström A (1963). Tooth morphology as a basis for distinguishing monozygotic and dizygotic twins. *Am J Hum Genet* 15:34-43.

Markovic M (1982). Hypodontia in twins. *Swed Dent J* (Suppl)15:153-162.

Markovic MD (1992). At the crossroads of oral facial genetics. *Eur J Orthod* 14:469-481.

McEwen JE, Boyer JT, Sun KY (2013). Evolving approaches to the ethical management of genomic data. *Trends Genet* 29:375-82.

Mizoguchi Y (1977). Genetic variability of permanent tooth crowns as ascertained from twin data. *J Anthrop Soc Nippon* 85:301-309.

Mulick JF (1965). An investigation of craniofacial asymmetry using the serial twin-study method. *Am J Orthod* 51:112-129.

Nakata M (1985). Twin studies in craniofacial genetics: a review. *Acta Genet Med Gemellol* 34:1-14.

Nakata M, Yu PL, Davis B, Nance WE (1973). The use of genetic data in the prediction of craniofacial dimensions. *Am J Orthod* 63:471-480.

Nakata M, Yu PL, Davis B, Nance WE (1974). Genetic determinants of cranio-facial morphology: a twin study. *Ann J Hum Genet* 37:431-443.

Neale MC (1995). *Mx: statistical modeling*, 3rd edn. Virginia: Virginia Commonwealth University.

Newman HH (1923). *The physiology of twinning*. Chicago: University of Chicago Press.

Newman HH (1928a). Studies of human twins. I. Methods of diagnosing monozygotic and dizygotic twins. *Biol Bull* 55:283-297.

Newman HH (1928b). Studies of human twins. II. Asymmetry reversal, of mirror imaging in identical twins. *Biol Bull* 55:298-315.

Newman HH (1930). Identical twins reared apart. *Eugen Rev* 22:29-34.

Newman HH (1934). Mental and physical traits of identical twins reared apart. Case I. Twins 'A' and 'O'. *J Hered* 25:49-64.

Newman HH, Freeman FN, Holzinger KJ (1937). *Twins: a study of heredity and environment*. Chicago: University of Chicago Press.

Nyström M, Ranta R (1988). Dental age and asymmetry in the formation of mandibular teeth in twins concordant or discordant for oral clefts. *Scand J Dent Res* 96:393-398.

Osborne RH (1961). Applications of twin studies to dental research. In: *Genetics and Dental Health*. Witkop C Jr, editor. New York: McGraw-Hill, pp. 79-91.

Osborne RH, De George FV (1959). *Genetic basis of morphological variation: an evaluation and application of the twin study method*. Cambridge: Harvard University Press.

Osborne RH, Horowitz SL, De George FV (1958). Genetic variation in tooth dimensions: a twin study of the permanent anterior teeth. *Am J Hum Genet* 10:350-356.

Peck S, Will LA (2004). In Memoriam: Coenraad F. A. Moorrees, 1916-2003. *Am J Orthod Dentofacial Orthop* 125:396-398.

Pillas D, Hoggart CJ, Evans DM, O'Reilly PF, Sipilä K, Lähdesmäki R, et al. (2010). Genome-wide association study reveals multiple loci associated with primary tooth development during infancy. *PloS Genet* 6:e1000856 doi:10.1371/journal.pgen.1000856. Accessed 19 May 2015.

Potter RH, Nance WE (1976). A twin study of dental dimension. I. Discordance, asymmetry, and mirror imagery. *Am J Phys Anthropol* 44:391-395.

Potter RH, Nance WE, Yu PL, Davis WB (1976). A twin study of dental dimension. II. Independent genetic determinants. *Am J Phys Anthrop* 44:397-412.

Rebich T, Markovic M (1976). Inheritance of tooth dimension: a quantitative genetic study. 52nd Congress June 28-Jul 2, *Trans Europ Orthod Soc*: 59-70.

Ribeiro DC, Brook AH, Hughes TE, Sampson WJ, Townsend GC (2013). Intrauterine hormone effects on tooth dimensions. *J Dent Res* 92:425-431.

Shapiro BL (1969). A twin study of palatal dimensions partitioning genetic and environmental contributions to variability. *Angle Orthod* 39:139-151.

Siemens HW (1927). The diagnosis of identity in twins. *J Hered* 18:201-209.

Siemens HW, Hunold X (1924). Zwillingspathologische Untersuchungen der Mundhöhle. *Arch Dermatol Syph* 147:409-423.

Sognnaes RF, Rawson RD, Gratt BM, Nguyen NBT (1982). Computer comparison of bitemark patterns in identical twins. *J Am Dent Assoc* 105:449-451.

Staley RN, Green LJ (1971). Bilateral asymmetry in tooth cusp occurrence in human monozygotic twins, dizygotic twins, and nontwins. *J Dent Res* 50:83-89.

Staley RN, Greene LJ (1974). Types of tooth cusp occurrence asymmetry in human monozygotic and dizygotic twins. *Am J Phys Anthropol* 40:187-195.

Su C-Y, Corby PM, Elliot MA, Studen-Pavlovich DA, Ranalli DN, Rosa B, et al. (2008). Inheritance of occlusal topography: a twin study. *Eur Arch Paediatr Dent* 9:19-24.

Tangchaitrong K, Messer LB, Thomas CDL, Townsend GC (2000). Fourier analysis of facial profiles of young twins. *Am J Phys Anthropol* 113:369-379.

Thesleff I (2006). The genetic basis of tooth development and dental defects. *Am J Med Genet A* 140:2530-2535.

Townsend GC, Martin NG (1992). Fitting genetic models to Carabelli trait data in South Australian twins. *J Dent Res* 71:403-409.

Townsend G, Richards L, Hughes T (2003). Molar intercuspal dimensions: genetic input to phenotypic variation. *J Dent Res* 82:350-355.

Townsend GC, Corruccini RS, Richards LC, Brown T (1988). Genetic and environmental determinants of dental occlusal variation in South Australian twins. *Aust Orthod J* 10:231-235.

van Dongen J, Slagboom PE, Draisma HHM, Martin NG, Boomsma DI (2012). The continuing value of twin studies in the omics era. *Nat Rev Genet* 13:640-653.

Chapter Four

COHORT 1: TEETH AND FACES OF SOUTH AUSTRALIAN TEENAGE TWINS

Introduction

There is an interesting lineage of researchers who influenced Grant Townsend and contributed directly or indirectly to the establishment of the three major studies of Australian twins and their families at the Adelaide Dental School. These studies commenced in 1983 and still continue today.

Townsend studied the subject 'Genetics and Human Variation IH' presented by Professor John Henry Bennett from the Department of Genetics at the University of Adelaide in 1973. This was part of his Honours year, referred to as a BScDent (Hons) degree. This subject included a practical component which involved Nick Martin as a tutor in the laboratory. Another member of the staff in the Department of Genetics at that time was Dr George Mayo, who was more than happy to answer questions about genetic aspects of dentistry and to help subsequently with any issues that arose in writing up papers from Townsend's PhD (Figure 4.1). Nick Martin has continued to be a magnificent supporter of the Adelaide Dental School twin studies over the past thirty-five years, always prepared to provide advice and to encourage and challenge us to 'push back the frontiers of knowledge'.

JH Bennett subsequently put together the combined works of Sir Ronald Fisher, who spent time in Adelaide during the 1960s. Fisher was a mentor to Kenneth Mather and John Jinks, who supervised Lindon Eaves's PhD; and Eaves, in turn, was a supervisor of Nick Martin's PhD.

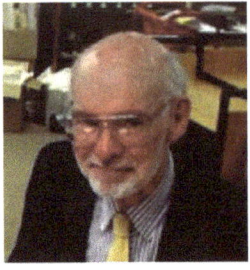 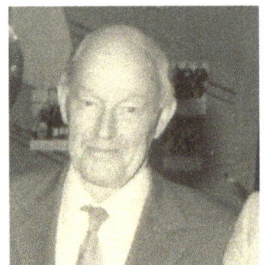 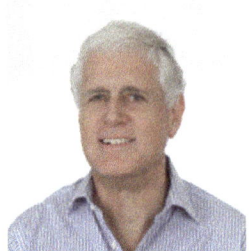

Figure 4.1
John Henry Bennett, George Elton Mayo and Nick Gordon Martin.

After being appointed to the academic staff of the Adelaide Dental School in 1977, Townsend and his PhD supervisor, Professor Tasman Brown, published some papers presenting the main findings of the thesis entitled *Tooth size variability in Australian Aboriginals: a descriptive and genetic study* (Townsend and Brown, 1978a,b; Townsend, 1978; Brown and Townsend, 1979; Townsend and Brown, 1979a,b). Townsend was well aware of the ongoing importance of the records collected in the 1950s and 1960s during the longitudinal growth study of Aboriginal Australians living at Yuendumu in the Northern Territory (Brown et al., 2011). He was keen to establish another ongoing study that would enable questions about the genetic basis of dental development and morphology to be further addressed, and he realised the potential of studying twins.

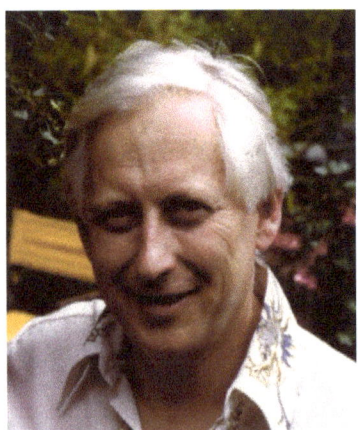

Figure 4.2
Tasman Brown.

Cohort 1: Teeth and faces of South Australian teenage twins

In November 1982, in collaboration with Nick Martin, who was with the Australian Twin Registry at the time, detailed planning for examination of the first cohort of South Australian twins began. This study drew heavily on the classical twin model, where comparisons are made between pairs of monozygotic and dizygotic twins to unravel the influences of genetic and environmental factors on observed variability of features. However, with the development around that time of more sophisticated statistical methods of genetic modelling, together with a growing appreciation of the unique nature of the twinning process, a clearer insight into the causes of non-genetic variability in twins was also beginning to emerge.

Cohort 1 (April 1983)

The general aim of this first study (now referred to as Cohort 1) was to estimate the relative contributions of genetic and non-genetic factors to observed variation in the teeth and faces of South Australian twins. It was hypothesised that there would be a strong genetic influence on variation observed in the dentition and facial structures, but that non-genetic (environmental) influences acting during pre- and postnatal development would also be important contributors to observed variability. Specifically, it was aimed to compare variability, including asymmetry, in different features of the teeth and dental arches in monozygotic and dizygotic twins, and also in singleton groups. It was also aimed to quantify and compare facial morphology, particularly asymmetry, in twins using stereophotogrammetric and computer-based techniques for the analysis of data in three dimensions.

This was the first study of the teeth and faces of twins using techniques such as stereophotogrammetry and computer modelling to be undertaken in Australia and one of the first in the world. It was hoped that when the collection of twin material was complete, there would be a unique resource available in Adelaide which would attract local and overseas researchers for years to come, in a similar manner to the Yuendumu material. Indeed, this has occurred, with a stream of researchers continuing to visit the Adelaide Dental School to examine the material.

The dentition provides an excellent model system, not only to study the genetic basis of craniofacial development, but also to investigate some of the questions of altered laterality (sidedness) associated with the twinning process. As we explained in Chapter One, teeth are particularly suitable for genetic studies because their final crown morphology is determined well before they emerge into the mouth, and they then remain stable, apart from the effects of wear or dental restorative procedures. Furthermore, embryological development of the dentition extends from about four weeks in utero through a series of recognisable stages of morphogenesis, differentiation, calcification and emergence until around twenty-one years postnatally. The teeth can therefore serve as a model system for studying the nature and timing of developmental disturbances that occur from early in life until after adolescence. The bilateral arrangement of the teeth also enables comparisons to be made of the size and shape of corresponding teeth on the right and left sides of the dental arches. This provides insights into questions of symmetry and asymmetry.

It was felt that combining the unique features of the dentition with the twinning process should prove to be a very fruitful avenue for research. Furthermore, it was considered that this type of research would have important implications, not only in clarifying the relative contributions of genetic and environmental influences to normal variation in dental and facial structures, but also in providing a rational approach to the prevention of disharmonies in the system. The studies that were planned aimed to provide insights into early developmental events in twinning, including the determination of body symmetry and the fascinating phenomenon of mirror imaging, where one member of a twin pair can mirror the other for one or more features.

Methodology and data acquisition

The first study of twins was limited mainly to teenage twins living in Adelaide. By the ages of 12 to 13 years, most children have all of their permanent teeth, except the third molars (or wisdom teeth). It was felt that this age group would be prepared to participate in a study that would involve dental examinations and obtaining dental impressions, as well as the donation of a blood sample to confirm zygosity.

In setting up the study, close liaison was maintained with the Australian Twin Registry in Melbourne, where a large database had been compiled of the names of twins and their families interested in participating in research projects. Letters inviting participation in the study were sent out to families of twins, and approximately 50 per cent of those contacted agreed to participate. The study was approved by the Research Advisory Committee of the Australian NHMRC Twin Registry, the Research Review Committee of the Royal Adelaide Hospital, and the

Cohort 1: Teeth and faces of South Australian teenage twins

Ethics Committee of the University of Adelaide. The NHMRC guidelines on human experimentation were followed.

The study involved examinations of the twins in the Adelaide Dental School. All of the participants were volunteers and were able to withdraw from the study at any time. There was no experimentation carried out in the strict sense, as the study only involved making observations and obtaining records from the participants. Apart from direct examination of the teeth and oral structures, records collected included dental impressions from which dental casts were constructed, stereophotographs of the face, extra-oral and intra-oral colour photographs of the face and teeth, and blood samples for zygosity determination.

The examinations took about forty-five minutes for each pair of twins, and often over twelve pairs of twins and their siblings would be seen each day. Other family members were also examined if they were agreeable. Colgate, a well-known company which produces various dental products including toothpaste and toothbrushes, was happy to offer its products to be included in special 'show bags' for the participants. Indeed, Colgate continues to support our research and we are extremely grateful for their ongoing generosity. We had arranged for a staff member from the Institute of Medical and Veterinary Science (IMVS) to come over to the Dental School (which is located next door) to obtain blood samples of the twins for zygosity testing. Ted Wild fulfilled this role very ably for many years and then, later, the twins would walk across to the IMVS building to be seen there.

It was decided to also record fingerprints and palm-prints from the twins. Dermatoglyphics, or the study of fingerprints, is a recognised area in physical anthropology and there have been many studies of fingerprint patterns in twins. These studies have confirmed that there is a strong genetic contribution to variation in the pattern of fingerprints on each finger. However, there were no published studies aimed at finding out whether there were common genetic factors influencing the shape of the teeth and the shape or pattern of fingerprints within individuals. Given that teeth and fingerprints are both derived from an interaction between epithelial tissue and mesenchymal tissue during development, it seemed that there could be common controlling mechanisms operating on both features. Furthermore, the arrangement of the fingers, with five on each hand, provides an opportunity to compare the expression of the patterns between fingers on one hand and between corresponding fingers on opposite hands. The dentition provides

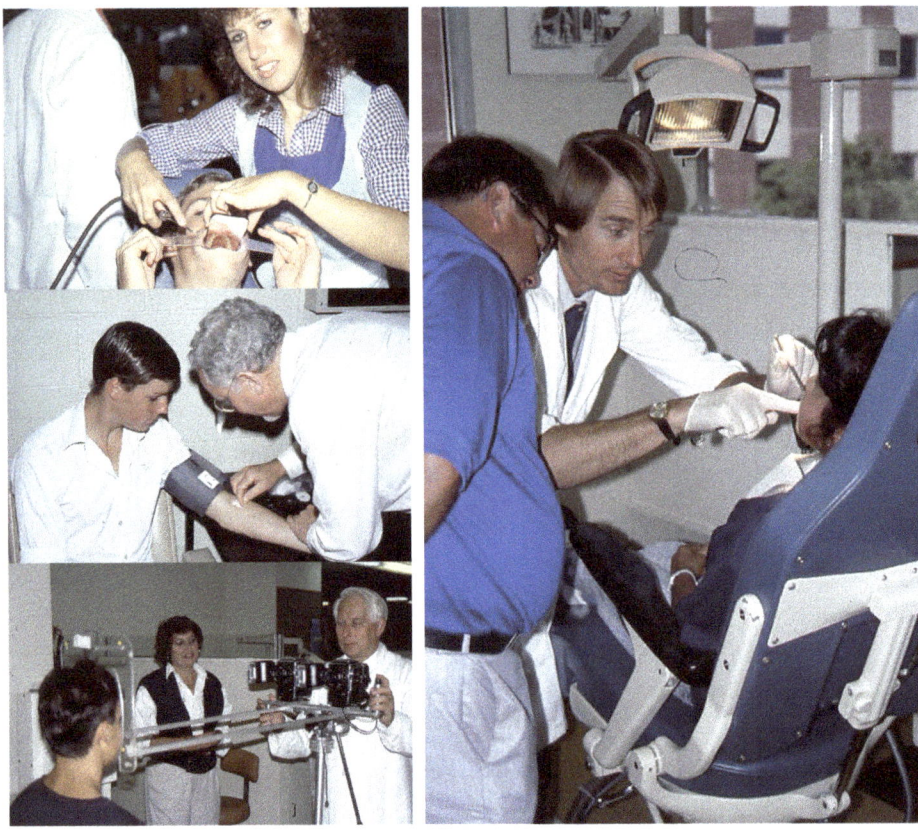

Figure 4.3
The team at work obtaining photographs of teeth, dental impressions, blood samples for zygosity determination and facial stereophotographs.

similar opportunities to compare the size and shape of different teeth within the same dental arch — for example, it is possible to compare the first molar with the second molar, as well as to make comparisons between corresponding teeth on opposite sides of the dental arch or in opposing arches. This is an area of research that we are currently exploring. Interestingly, there have been some recent reports of associations between different patterns of fingerprints and susceptibility to dental decay (Abhilash et al., 2012).

In collaboration with Dr David Hay, at that time in the Department of Genetics and Human Variation at La Trobe University, fingerprints and palm-prints were also collected (Figure 4.4), as well as information relating to laterality

Cohort 1: Teeth and faces of South Australian teenage twins

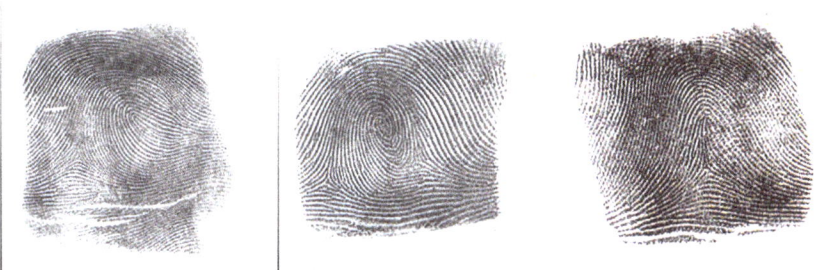

Figure 4.4
Examples of fingerprint patterns: a loop, a whorl and a tented arch (left to right).

(for example, handedness, foot dominance and eye dominance). Information about birthweights and lengths of the twins was also gathered, as well as medical histories.

With the assistance of Professor Bhim S Savara, a visiting Fulbright scholar in 1983, a procedure for obtaining facial stereophotographs of the twins was developed using two Hasselblad cameras mounted on a special frame for photogrammetric accuracy (Figure 4.5).

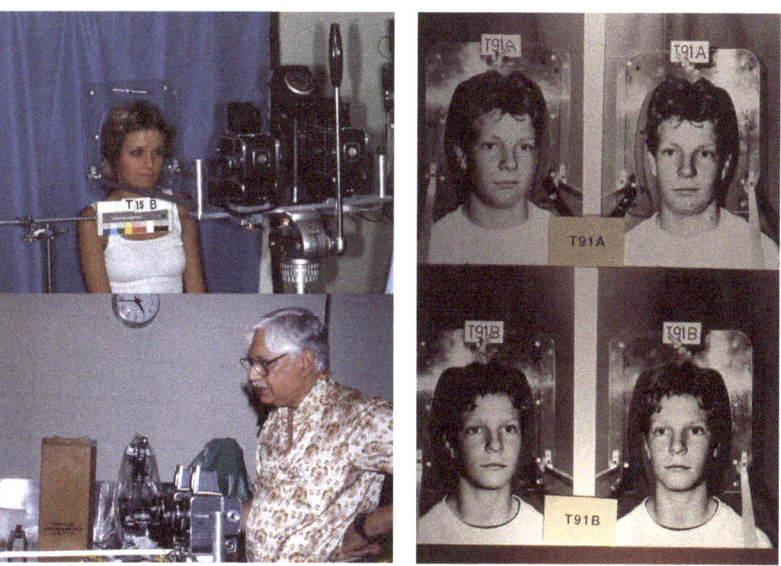

Figure 4.5
The stereophotographic set-up with Bhim Savara and an example of stereophotographs of a pair of monozygotic twins.

George Travan was appointed as a Research Officer in the Adelaide School of Dentistry in 1984 (Figure 4.6). His background in computer science was invaluable for the development of the software, and he also established an excellent liaison with the Faculty of Engineering. This enabled access to computer packages that were very advanced for the time and that ran on the University's VAX system, enabling manipulation of three-dimensional (3D) data, including the display and modelling of complex surfaces such as those characterising the human face. With the assistance of scientists from different South Australian Government departments, Travan produced machine-milled facial models. These were visually striking, and the approaches developed were subsequently applied by surgeons in the Australian Craniofacial Unit at the Adelaide Women's and Children's Hospital.

This facial mapping procedure was similar to that used to survey contour maps, and it quantified the face in three dimensions, with contour lines at regular intervals representing the third dimension. Output in the form of 3D co-ordinates, stored on magnetic tape in those days, could then be transferred to the mainframe computer at the University of Adelaide for further processing. Tasman Brown and George Travan then developed custom-made software to enable the facial images to be generated by the computer and displayed in any orientation.

When a Sun 3/60 workstation was installed in our own laboratory, we were able to better process the large data sets that we were generating, particularly in

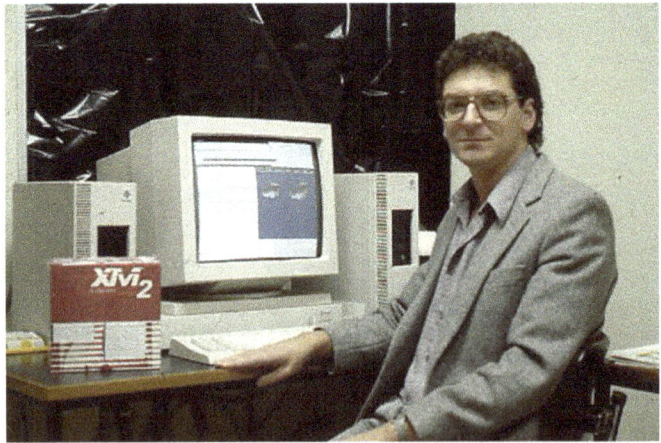

Figure 4.6
George Travan with his SUN workstation.

Cohort 1: Teeth and faces of South Australian teenage twins

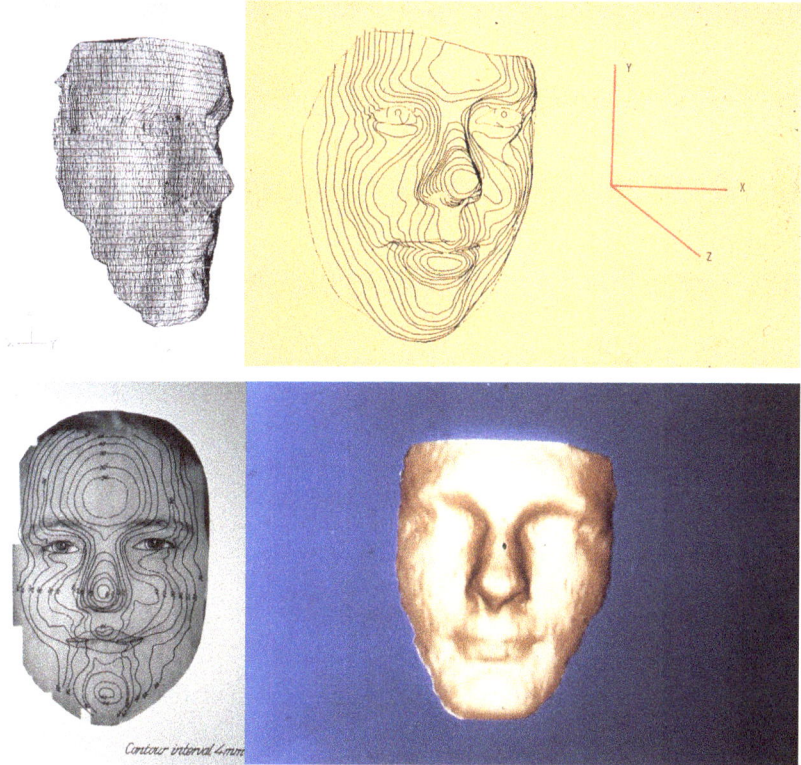

Figure 4.7
Examples of early attempts to produce contour maps and wireframe and solid models of twins' faces.

relation to graphic representations. Codenamed 'Ferrari' by the manufacturers, the Sun workstation was considered to be a very powerful computer at this time. By today's standards, however, its specifications would be surpassed by a smartphone!

For the genetic analysis of the faces of twins, we took the stereopairs obtained from the two Hasselblad cameras and positioned them in a Wild-Leitz stereoviewer. Reference points and principal points were marked on the left and right images. The films were then positioned on a Summagraphics digitiser in appropriate orientation, and co-ordinates of each reference point were obtained on each left and right image (Figure 4.8). Software, developed from standard photogrammetric algorithms, allowed us to calculate the 3D co-ordinates of each point, taking into account scaling factors and the geometry of the photographic system. We selected reference points from those in common use in medicine and anthropology, representing anatomical

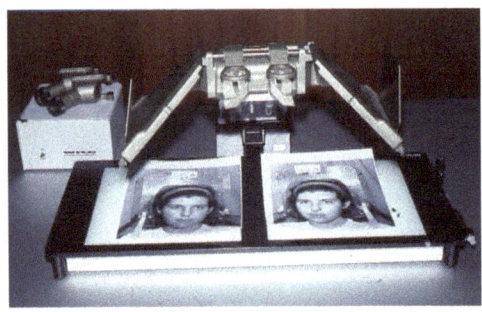
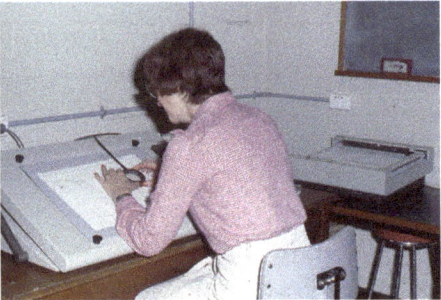

Figure 4.8
Stereoviewer for examining facial photographs and Wendy Schwerdt digitising.

features of the eyes, nose and mouth. There are obvious limitations with these types of soft tissue points, many of which are located in movable tissues, but the results of our replicability studies were encouraging.

Another piece of equipment that we thought was state-of-the-art in the 1980s was a set of digital callipers with specially sharpened tips that enabled us to measure the size of thousands of tooth crowns from the dental models that we had constructed (Figure 4.9). These callipers enabled measurements to be made to an accuracy of 0.1 mm and they were connected to an Apple IIc computer that was set up to enable measurements to be recorded rapidly and accurately in digital format. Although

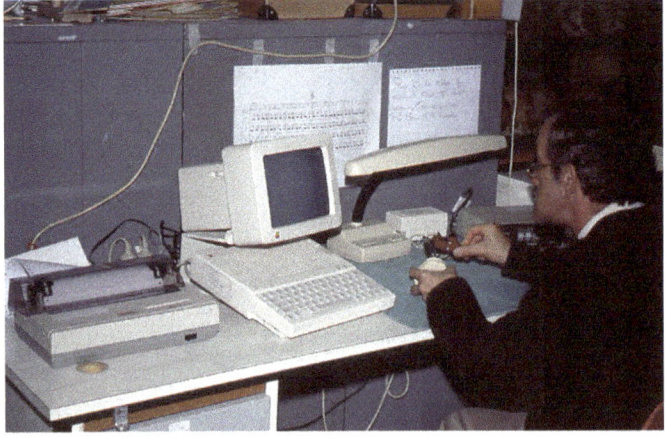

Figure 4.9
Jim Rogers measuring teeth with digital callipers connected to an Apple IIc computer.

callipers are still used by some researchers to record tooth size measurements, there is always a risk that the sharpened beaks of the callipers will scratch the dental models. For this reason, and coupled with the rapid developments in digital imaging, many studies of tooth size, including our own, are now based on obtaining indirect measurements from 2D or 3D digital images.

In collaboration with researchers from Nihon University at Matsudo in Japan, including Dr Mitsuo Sekikawa, we also applied techniques of Moiré photography to enable complex surfaces, such as dental crowns, to be imaged and then measured in 3D with an accuracy of 0.2 mm (Figure 4.10).

A number of developments for the analysis of twin data were being applied in the 1980s. The approach of Martin and Eaves from Birmingham (Martin et al., 1978) and also those of Christian and colleagues from Indiana (Christian, 1979) were used in Adelaide. The twin model computer programs developed by Christian, referred to as TANOVA and TWNAN, were adapted for use on the University's VAX computer and then tested and verified. These were the days when 'big jobs' like this had to be run on the University's central mainframe computer — how things have changed! Development of this software in Adelaide led to a very productive collaboration with Rob Corruccini (Figure 4.11) from Southern Illinois University, USA.

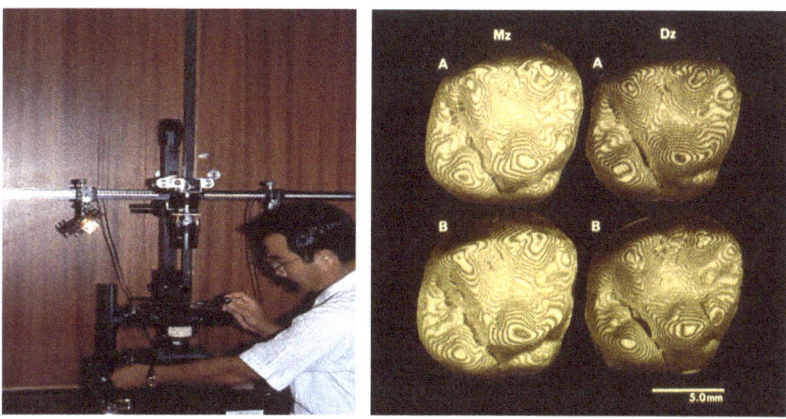

Figure 4.10
Mitsuo Sekikawa adjusting the Moiré equipment and the resultant images of permanent upper first molars from a pair of monozygotic (MZ) twins and a pair of dizygotic (DZ) twins. Images of teeth reproduced with permission of Nihon University Journal of Oral Science (copyright) (Sekikawa et al., 1989).

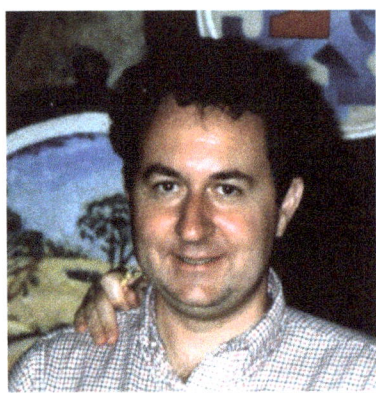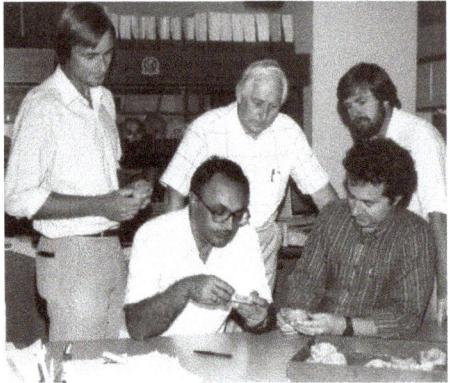

Figure 4.11
Rob Corruccini, and Rob with Samvit Kaul, Grant Townsend, Tasman Brown and Lindsay Richards.

Townsend met Corruccini at the VIIth International Symposium on Dental Morphology in Paris in 1986 (Russell et al., 1988). Corruccini had previously presented evidence that non-genetic factors, probably related to food consistency and chewing force, were likely to be important determinants in the development of dental occlusion — that is, the way the teeth fit together. He proposed that the increased frequency of malocclusion in modern human populations following industrialisation had occurred too rapidly to be explained in genetic terms and that it was more likely that this trend was related to the adoption of softer Western-style diets. During a period of sabbatical leave in Adelaide in 1987, Corruccini scored occlusal traits in the South Australian twin sample, using similar methods to those that he had applied to US and Indian samples. He made various observations and measurements from our dental models, and then the genetic analyses of Christian and colleagues were applied to the data. This research led to a paper published in the *Australian Orthodontic Journal* and another in *Human Biology* (Townsend et al., 1988a; Corruccini et al., 1990).

In 1986, Townsend also participated in the 5th International Congress on Twin Studies, in Amsterdam, the Netherlands. It was here that he met Charles (Chuck) Boklage and was fortunate enough to spend some time talking with him about twins and twinning, and listening to some of his ideas. Boklage has been a provocative figure in twin research for decades and the results of his research on tooth size in twins have served as an impetus for many of our projects in Adelaide. He recently published a book summarising his main findings entitled *How New Humans are Made*. It is a very stimulating read and poses many thought-provoking questions about the nature of the twinning process and the development of body symmetry (Boklage, 2010).

In the foreword to the papers inspired by an international workshop on twin methodology held in Belgium in 1987 and published in a special issue of the journal *Behavior Genetics*, Martin and colleagues pointed out that

> twin studies are growing larger and more complex every year as workers from a wide variety of biomedical and behavioural disciplines realize the power of twin designs. Yet many of these studies are analyzed in no more depth than could have been achieved in 1929 when Holzinger formulized the intuitive argument put forth by Galton in 1875. (Martin et al., 1989)

This statement was particularly relevant to twin studies of dental morphology which had been carried out in the past or were being carried out at the time, where the ultimate aim was merely to calculate values of heritability, usually without any attempt to provide error estimates. Martin's statement had a strong effect on our research group, and it was decided that the most up-to-date methods needed to be used when analysing our twin data.

Fitting genetic models to dental data from twins

In the early 1990s, with the help of Nick Martin, model-fitting approaches began to be applied to analyse our twin data. The software program for structural equation modelling, called LISREL, was used, along with its pre-processor, PRELIS. These programs were applied to both discrete and continuous data. At this point, structural equation models had been used for some time in the social and behavioural sciences, but they were only beginning to be used more widely in human genetics. Indeed, to our knowledge, we were the first group of dental researchers to apply these much more sophisticated types of genetic modelling to large sets of dento-facial data.

Until this time, many dental researchers had tended to concentrate on rarer Mendelian disorders rather than trying to analyse the more common, but complex, traits, such as tooth size and facial dimensions. Many of the variables that we planned to examine in our study did not display simple modes of inheritance — for example, autosomal dominant or recessive — but appeared to be modified to varying degrees by environmental factors. Indeed, many of the phenotypes of interest to oral health professionals, such as dental caries and periodontal disease, show multifactorial modes of inheritance, with genotypes responding to an array of environments. These phenotypes tend to show continuous distributions ranging from normal to abnormal in the extremes.

The shape-fitting algorithms that our group was using for comparisons of facial images between the twins also needed to be developed and implemented on our personal computers, the Sun system and the university's VAX computer. These programs enabled representations of the faces of monozygotic and dizygotic twins to be rotated and superimposed to highlight similarities and differences between co-twins, including evidence of mirror imaging (Figures 4.12 and 4.13).

An 'advanced' database system was also developed using SIR software to electronically store and access the twin records. This is essential in studies that generate large amounts of data. More recently, we have implemented a new relational database using a Microsoft Access front-end user interface and an MS SQL 2015 Server backend to store the data. Similar to the advances in computing technology mentioned above, this new system is several orders of magnitude more sophisticated than the original SIR system. It provides ease of data entry and access and has significant redundancy to ensure data are maintained with high fidelity in the event of a system failure. This is important, as funding bodies such as the NHMRC now have specific requirements for how funded medical research data are collected, stored, archived and, where necessary, disposed of, in line with ethical and privacy requirements. The University of Adelaide has also implemented a broad-based data repository to assist with reporting requirements, and our system will eventually send summary research data to this server.

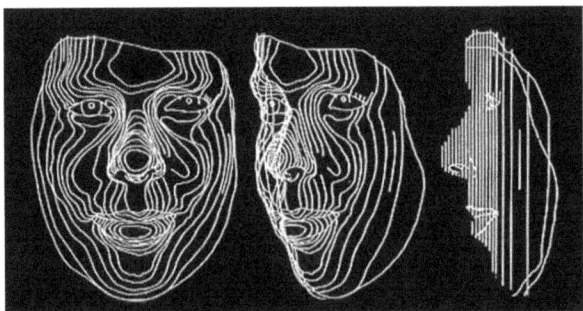

Figure 4.12
Contour maps of the face of a twin rotated from frontal to lateral views.

Cohort 1: Teeth and faces of South Australian teenage twins

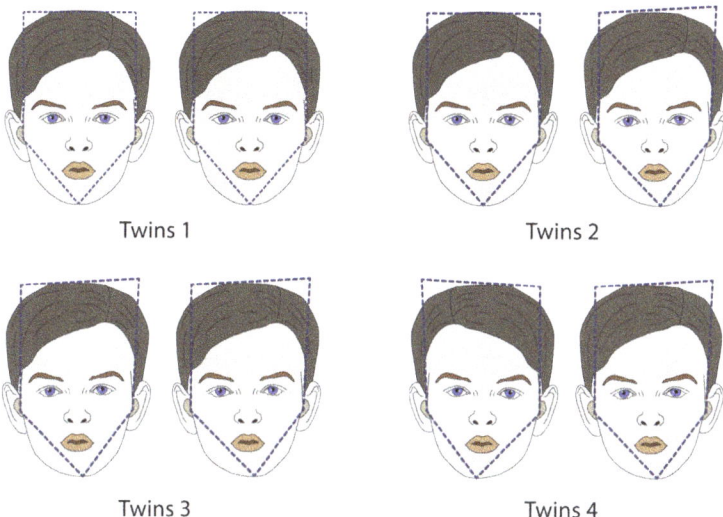

Figure 4.13
Theoretical combinations of facial asymmetry. Twins 1 — symmetry of both faces; Twins 2 — asymmetry in one face (in right facial image); Twins 3 — concordant asymmetry in both faces; and Twins 4 — discordant asymmetry of faces, with mirror imaging. Reproduced with permission of the Australian Dental Journal (Hughes et al., 2014).

Some of the variables studied in this first study included various features of the teeth such as the size of the dental crowns — for example, maximum mesiodistal and buccolingual crown diameters, as well as intercuspal distances. However, traditional measures of maximum tooth crown size provide little insight into the nature of dental crown shape. Some previous studies from our group had indicated that measurements based on the cusp tips would be more likely to provide biologically meaningful data, as these sites represent the sites of initial crown calcification (refer to Figure 1.5 in Chapter One).

One of the first morphological crown features studied was Carabelli trait. An example of its expression in the form of a large additional cusp on permanent maxillary first molars in a pair of monozygotic twins is provided in Figure 4.14. The heritability estimate for this feature was found to be very high, around 90 per cent, indicating that most of its variation could be accounted for by genetic factors.

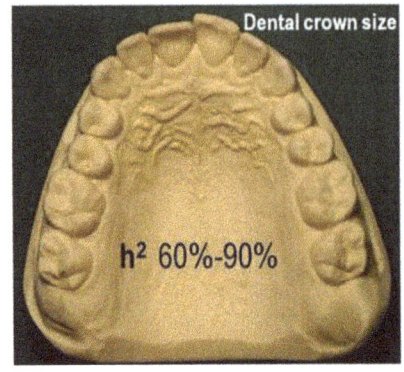
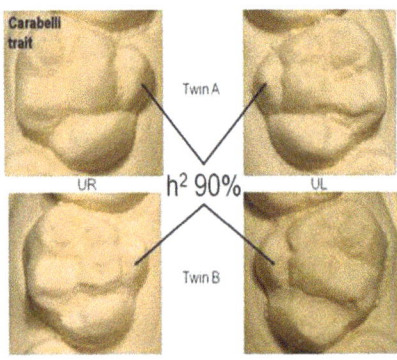
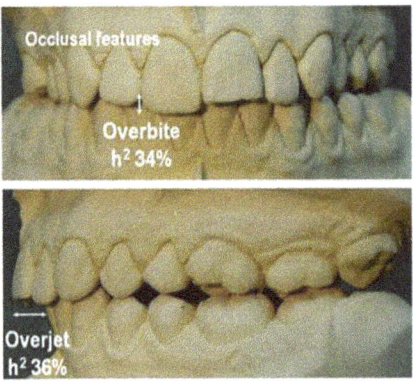

Figure 4.14
Estimates of heritability (h^2) for different dental features: dental crown size, Carabelli trait and anterior overbite and overjet. Values for heritability can range from 0 to 100 per cent (Townsend et al., 2012).

Cohort 1: Teeth and faces of South Australian teenage twins

By examining the mixed dentition of individuals and scoring the expression of features such as Carabelli trait on both primary and permanent teeth, it is possible to gain insight into both genetic and environmental influences on observed variation of teeth that have formed at different times. That is, such an examination provides something like a mini-longitudinal study of an individual based on a single dental model.

Apart from showing an example of Carabelli trait in a pair of monozygotic twins, Figure 4.14 also shows that the heritability estimates obtained for dental crown size have also been high, ranging from 60 per cent to 90 per cent. In contrast, estimates of heritability for some occlusal features, such as anterior overbite and overjet, have been low, indicating that non-genetic factors contribute significantly to observed variation.

On a side-note, it is rather exciting to realise that a pair of monozygotic twin boys, sons of one of a pair of monozygotic twin girls who participated in Cohort 1 at age 17 years, participated in Cohort 2. The boys are now adults in their mid-twenties and their parents are in their forties (Figure 4.15).

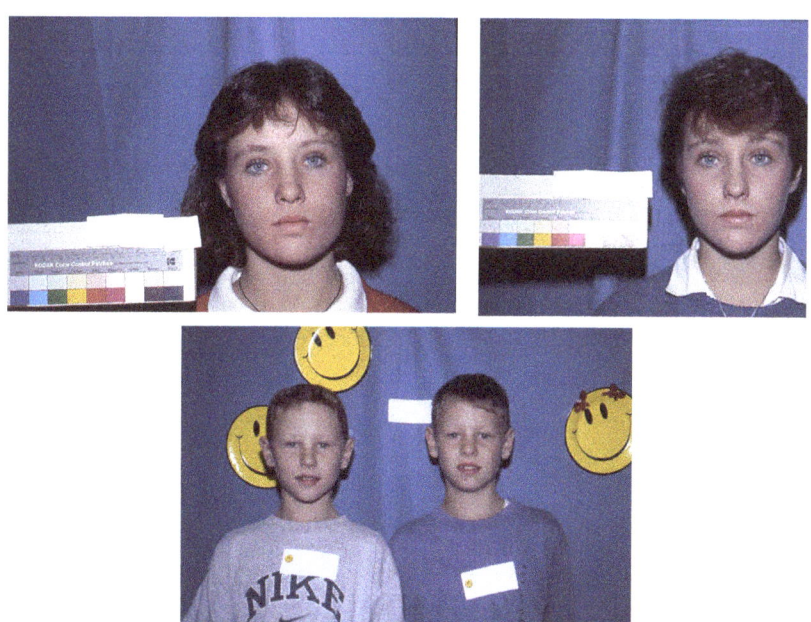

Figure 4.15
Two generations of twins who participated in Cohorts 1 and 2.

Some key findings of our studies involving Cohort 1

Some of the studies summarised below were untaken while we were involved in collecting data for Cohort 2 (described in the next chapter). However, they were based on data obtained from Cohort 1 and were related to the main aims of that study.

1. Using newer methods of analysis, our studies showed that previous estimates of heritability for tooth size were probably exaggerated because various assumptions of twin research had not been tested. Using a method for shape matching based on least squares fit of homologous co-ordinates (a statistical method of comparing two shapes represented by corresponding points), differences in facial asymmetry were detected between male and female dizygotic twins, and evidence of mirror imaging was noted in some monozygotic twin pairs (Townsend et al., 1986; Brown et al., 1992). This was one of the earliest applications of shape matching in this context and a precursor to the present-day geometric morphometric analyses that are being increasingly used in studies of evolution and development (Al-Shahrani et al., 2014).

2. It was shown that it is possible to determine the zygosity of twins very accurately by making comparisons of the appearance of their teeth. Only three pairs of twins from 120 pairs were 'misclassified' on the basis of dental morphology, all being classified as dizygotic whereas blood tests indicated that they were monozygotic (Townsend et al., 1988b). This finding has implications in the field of forensic odontology for identification of individuals from their teeth.

3. It was noted that there was a relatively small contribution of genetic factors to variation in some of the features that indicate how the upper and lower teeth fit together — for example, anterior overbite and overjet. This emphasises the importance of environmental influences on occlusal variation, a finding that has implications for the way in which orthodontists view the causes of malocclusions and, consequently, the way in which they may be prevented or treated (Townsend et al., 1988a; Corruccini et al., 1990).

4. It was noted that genetic factors play an important role in contributing to variation in dental arch shape but not to asymmetry in arch form

(Richards et al., 1990). This finding confirms the clinical impression that the symmetrical shapes of the dental arches are under strong genetic influence but that asymmetries are likely to be due to localised environmental effects, such as pressures from the tongue, lips and cheeks.

5. By fitting newly developed genetic models to data for Carabelli trait, a morphological feature that appears mainly on permanent upper first molars and primary upper second molars, values for heritability of around 90 per cent were found, suggesting that there is a very strong genetic influence of variation of this feature. This has important implications for anthropological studies that use dental features, such as Carabelli trait, to make inferences about affinities and migratory patterns of past and present human populations (Townsend and Martin, 1992).

6. Many examples of mirror imaging in the teeth and faces of twins in Cohort 1 have been noted, and approximately 30 per cent of monozygotic twins in the sample showed discordance for handedness, presumably reflecting differences in cerebral lateralisation. At the time that the study was performed, it was not possible to demonstrate any clear association between mirror imaging and chorion (foetal membrane) type of the twins, as ultrasound technology had not advanced to its present stage (Townsend et al., 1994).

7. A mathematical approach based on Fourier functions showed that there is a significant genetic contribution to variation in the convexity of the facial profile, facial height and facial depth. Variability in nose and lip morphology, however, appeared to be under stronger environmental influence (Vanco et al., 1995). These findings have significance for researchers in the field of craniofacial biology and for practising orthodontists.

8. A study of congenitally missing upper lateral incisors (agenesis) in our twin sample showed that the frequency was similar to singletons (around 2 per cent) and identified five pairs of monozygotic twins who displayed varying expressions of normal, small, peg-shaped and missing upper laterals. These findings were consistent with a multifactorial threshold model linking tooth size and number, as described initially by Brook

(1984). It was proposed that developmental influences were likely to modify the appearance of the lateral incisors in those monozygotic twin pairs whose genetic make-up placed them near the threshold for either having a lateral incisor or not (Townsend et al., 1995). This concept was expanded further in a later paper that is reported in Chapter Five.

9. Paula Dempsey completed her PhD entitled *The nature of genetic and environmental contributions to dental variation in twins and their families* in 1998. Her co-supervisors were Townsend and Martin. Several excellent papers arose from her research, which was one of the first comprehensive analyses of the human dentition based on sophisticated genetic modelling of data derived from a large sample of twins. By applying multivariate genetic modelling methods to tooth size data, it was possible to partition out the various sources of genetic and environmental variation in much greater detail than had been possible previously. This study revealed a strong contribution of additive genetic effects, as well as shared environmental influences and unique environmental effects. There also appeared to be symmetry of the genetic and environmental influences between right and left sides. Other papers based on Dempsey's research reported evidence of non-additive genetic effects on the canines, suggesting an important role for these teeth during human evolution. Common environmental effects were most strongly associated with the permanent first molars, indicating a possible role of the uterine environment in the determination of the size of these teeth (Dempsey et al., 1995; Dempsey et al., 1999a; Dempsey and Townsend, 2001). These findings have important implications for studies of human evolution and dental development.

10. Collaborative studies of facial asymmetry and attractiveness in our sample of twins with an American psychologist, the late Linda Mealey, showed that the more symmetric twin of a pair was consistently rated as more attractive, and that the magnitude of the difference between twins in perceived attractiveness was directly related to the magnitude of the perceived difference in symmetry. These results support the evolutionary model of mate choice and also the medical model of fluctuating asymmetry as an indicator of developmental health. This work has been cited widely and shows how studies of teeth and faces can have very wide-

ranging applications and significance (Mealey et al., 1999, Mealey and Townsend, 1999).

11. There are several different twin models that can be used for research purposes. One involves studying opposite-sex dizygotic twin pairs. We showed, for the first time, that the females from opposite-sex dizygotic twin pairs had larger teeth than the females from either dizygotic same-sex twin pairs or monozygotic twin pairs. This study provided support for the Twin Testosterone Transfer (TTT) hypothesis, which proposes that androgens can diffuse from a male to a female foetus in utero, influencing behavioural and morphological traits (Dempsey et al., 1999b). A more recent study by Daniela Ribeiro, which formed part of her PhD thesis, provided further support for the TTT hypothesis (Ribeiro et al., 2013).

12. In another study, we hypothesised that intercuspal distances of human molar teeth would show greater phenotypic variation but lower heritabilities (that is, the contribution of genetic factors to observed variation) than traditional overall crown measures (that is, maximum mesiodistal and buccolingual crown diameters). Our findings supported this hypothesis and were, therefore, consistent with substantial epigenetic influence on the progressive folding of the internal enamel epithelium of developing molar teeth, following the formation of the primary and secondary enamel knots. The significance of these findings was that they helped to draw together the results of molecular biologists and dental anthropologists in providing a more comprehensive explanation of the developmental events that lead to the phenotypic appearance of fully formed teeth (Townsend et al., 2003).

13. Although our studies of twins have focused on teeth and faces, we have also collected data on handedness, and our findings have been included in two publications (Dempsey et al., 1999c; Medland et al., 2009). In the earlier one of these papers, which was based entirely on our Australian sample, it was shown that the frequency of non-right-handedness was elevated in twins of all zygosities (12 to 23 per cent) compared with frequencies reported for the general population (around 10 per cent). In this study, no significant associations were found between handedness and sex, or zygosity, or birth order or birthweight. There was no evidence for

a significant genetic effect on handedness or for birth factors. However, there is always an issue of statistical power in these types of studies — that is, whether the sample sizes are large enough to show a significant effect. The later study included many twin studies from all around the world, with a total sample of 54 270 individuals and 25 732 families. Interestingly, there was no evidence of hormonal effects, mirror imaging or twin specific effects in this very large sample. Furthermore, there were no differences in the prevalence of non-right-handedness between zygosity groups or between twins and their singleton siblings. There was evidence that additive genetic effects contributed to about 25 per cent of the observed variation in handedness, with the rest due to non-shared environmental influences.

REFERENCES

Abhilash PR, Divyashree R, Patil SG, Gupta M, Chandrasekar T, Karthikeyan R (2012). Dermatoglyphics in patients with dental caries: a study on 1250 individuals. *J Contemp Dent Pract* 13:266-274.

Al-Shahrani I, Dirks W, Jepson N, Khalaf K (2014). 3D-Geomorphometrics tooth shape analysis in hypondontia. *Front Physiol.* 5:154. doi:10.3389/fphys.2014.00154 Accessed 21 May 2015.

Boklage CE (2010). *How new humans are made.* Singapore: World Scientific Publishing Co. Pte. Ltd.

Brook AH (1984). A unifying aetiological explanation for anomalies of human tooth number and size. *Arch Oral Biol* 29:373-378.

Brown T, Townsend G (1979). Sex determination by single and multiple tooth measurements. In: *Occasional Papers in Human Biology 1*. Canberra: Australian Institute of Aboriginal Studies, pp. 1-16,

Brown T, Townsend GC, Pinkerton SK, Rogers JR (2011). *Yuendumu: legacy of a longitudinal growth study in Central Australia*. Adelaide: University of Adelaide Press.

Brown T, Townsend GC, Richards LC, Travan GR, Pinkerton SK (1992). Facial symmetry and mirror imaging in South Australian twins. In: *Craniofacial Variation in Pacific Populations*. Brown T, Molnar S, editors. Adelaide: Anthropology and Genetics Laboratory, The University of Adelaide, pp. 79-98.

Christian JC (1979). Testing twin means and estimating genetic variance: basic methodology for the analysis of quantitative twin data. *Acta Genet Med Gemellol* 28:35-40.

Corruccini RS, Townsend GC, Richards LC, Brown T (1990). Genetic and environmental determinants of dental occlusal variation in twins of different nationalities. *Hum Biol* 62:353-367.

Dempsey PJ, Townsend GC (2001). Genetic and environmental contributions to variation in human tooth size. *Heredity* 86:685-693.

Dempsey PJ, Townsend GC, Martin NG (1999a). Insights into the genetic basis of human dental variation from statistical modelling analyses. *Perspec Hum Biol* 4(3):9-17.

Dempsey PJ, Townsend GC, Richards LC (1999b). Increased tooth crown size in females with twin brothers: evidence for hormonal diffusion between human twins in utero. *Am J Hum Biol* 11:577-586.

Dempsey P, Schwerdt W, Townsend G, Richards L (1999c). Handedness in twins: the search for genetic and environmental causes. *Perspec Hum Biol* 4(3):37-44.

Dempsey PJ, Townsend GC, Martin NG, Neale MC (1995). Genetic covariance structure of incisor crown size in twins. *J Dent Res* 74:1389-1398.

Hughes TE, Townsend GC, Pinkerton SK, Bockmann MR, Seow WK, Brook AH, et al. (2014). The teeth and faces of twins: providing insights into dentofacial development and oral health for practising oral health professionals. *Aust Dent J* 59 (1 Suppl):101-116.

Martin NG, Boomsma DI, Neale MC (1989). Foreword. *Behav Genet* 19:5-7.

Martin NG, Eaves LJ, Kearsey MJ, Davies P (1978). The power of the classical twin study. *Heredity* 40:97-116.

Mealey L, Townsend GC (1999). The role of fluctuating asymmetry on judgements of physical attractiveness: a monozygotic co-twin comparison. *Perspec Hum Biol* 4(1):219-224.

Mealey L, Bridgstock R, Townsend GC (1999). Symmetry and perceived facial attractiveness: a monozygotic co-twin comparison. *J Pers Soc Psychol* 76:151-158.

Medland SE, Duffy DL, Wright MJ, Geffen GM, Hay DA, Levy F, et al. (2009). Genetic influences on handedness: data from 25,732 Australian and Dutch twin families. *Neuropsychologia* 47:330-337.

Ribeiro DC, Brook AH, Hughes TE, Sampson WJ, Townsend GC (2013). Intrauterine hormone effects on tooth dimensions. *J Dent Res* 92:425-431.

Richards LC, Townsend GC, Brown T, Burgess VB (1990). Dental arch morphology in South Australian twins. *Arch Oral Biol* 35:983-989.

Russell DE, Santoro J-P, Sigogneau-Russell D (1988). *Teeth revisited: Proceedings of the VIIth International Symposium on Dental Morphology.* Mémoires du

Muséum National D'Histoire Naturelle, Sciences de la Terre, Tome 53. Paris: Éditions du Muséum Paris.

Sekikawa M, Namuri T, Kanazawa E, Ozaki T, Richards LC, Townsend GC et al. (1989). Three-dimensional measurement of the maxillary first molar in Australian Whites. *Nihon Univ J Oral Sci* 15:457-464.

Townsend G (1978). Genetics of tooth size. *Aust Orthodont J* 5:142-147.

Townsend G, Bockmann M, Hughes T, Mihailidis S, Seow WK, Brook A (2012). New approaches to dental anthropology based on the study of twins. In: *New Directions in Dental Anthropology: paradigms, methodologies and outcomes.* Townsend G, Kanazawa E, Takayama H, editors. Adelaide: University of Adelaide Press, pp. 10-21.

Townsend GC, Brown T (1978a). Inheritance of tooth size in Australian Aboriginals. *Am J Phys Anthropol* 48:305-314.

Townsend GC, Brown T (1978b). Heritability of permanent tooth size. *Am J Phys Anthropol* 49:497-504.

Townsend GC, Brown T (1979a). Family studies of tooth size factors in the permanent dentition. *Am J Phys Anthropol* 50:183-190.

Townsend G, Brown T (1979b). Tooth size characteristics of Australian Aborigines. *Occasional papers in Human Biology 1.* Canberra: Australian Institute of Aboriginal Studies, pp. 17-38.

Townsend GC, Brown T, Richards LC, Rogers JR, Pinkerton SK, Travan GR et al. (1986). Metric analyses of the teeth and faces of South Australian twins. *Acta Genet Med Gemellol* 35:179-192.

Townsend GC, Corruccini RS, Richards LC, Brown T (1988a). Genetic and environmental determinants of dental occlusion variation in South Australian twins. *Aust Orthod J* 10:231-235.

Townsend GC, Richards LC, Brown T, Burgess VB (1988b). Twin zygosity determination on the basis of dental morphology. *J Forensic Odontostomatol* 6:1-15.

Townsend GC, Martin NG (1992). Fitting genetic models to Carabelli trait data in South Australian twins. *J Dent Res* 71:403-409.

Townsend G, Richards L, Brown T, Pinkerton S (1994). Mirror imaging in twins: some dental examples. *Dent Anthropol News* 9:2-5.

Townsend G, Richards L, Hughes T (2003). Molar intercuspal dimensions: genetic input to phenotypic variation. *J Dent Res* 82:350-355.

Townsend G, Rogers J, Richards L, Brown T (1995). Agenesis of permanent maxillary lateral incisors in South Australian twins. *Aust Dent J* 40:186-192.

Vanco C, Kasai K, Sergi R, Richards LC, Townsend GC (1995). Genetic and environmental influences on facial profile. *Aust Dent J* 40:104-109.

Chapter Five

COHORT 2 – A LONGITUDINAL STUDY OF DENTAL AND FACIAL DEVELOPMENT IN AUSTRALIAN TWINS AND THEIR FAMILIES

INTRODUCTION

In 1994 the Craniofacial Biology Group decided that it would be valuable to carry out a comprehensive study of dental and facial development and morphology in young twins in the 4-6-year-old age interval to supplement previous studies of teenage twins. At that time, there had been no detailed studies of the teeth or faces of young twins with primary (deciduous) teeth. It was also not known whether special features of the twinning process affected dental and facial features of young twins. It was planned, if funding allowed, to re-examine these twins again around the ages of 9 to 11 years and then at around 12 to 14 years of age. This would then become one of the few longitudinal studies of twins focusing on teeth and faces to be carried out worldwide.

The aim in setting up this study of young twins, who are now referred to as Cohort 2, was to extend the use of newly developed methods of genetic model-fitting to data obtained from teeth and faces of both monozygotic and dizygotic twins, so that we could clarify in more detail than previously the roles of genetic and environmental determinants on observed variation. We also aimed to compare the expression of bilateral dental and facial features on the right and left sides, in both twins and singletons, to see the extent to which the twinning process affects the determination of body symmetry. This included our desire to explore more fully the fascinating phenomenon of mirror imaging, where one twin of a pair mirrors the other for one or more features.

As has been emphasised earlier, the primary teeth provide an excellent model system to study genetic aspects of dental and facial development. They also have advantages for investigating some of the questions relating to observed developmental differences between dental and facial features on the right and left sides (disturbed laterality) thought to be associated with the twinning process.

Most of the development of the primary tooth crowns occurs between approximately four weeks in utero and birth, with all the crowns being completely formed by around twelve months postnatally. This developmental span enables an assessment of how various pre- and perinatal factors, such as maternal health, smoking and alcohol consumption, placenta type and birth weight, might influence dental structures.

Once the primary teeth have emerged into the oral cavity, their crowns do not change in size or shape, apart from due to the effects of wear, disease or restorative procedures. The bilateral arrangement of teeth within the dental arches also enables comparisons to be made of the size and morphology of corresponding teeth on the right and left sides, providing insight into questions of symmetry and asymmetry.

The high standard of oral health in South Australian children during the 1990s meant that most of the children in the 4-6-year-old age range had full primary dentitions with very few restorations. Interestingly, this has changed over the past twenty years, with nearly half of Australian children in the 5-6-year-old age bracket now having a history of dental decay affecting their primary teeth. Similarly, nearly half of Australian 12-year-olds now have a history of decay in their permanent teeth. Of considerable concern is that those children from the lowest socioeconomic areas have about 70 per cent more dental decay than those from the highest socioeconomic regions of Australia (Ha et al., 2011). The reasons for this recent increase in decay in Australian children are likely to include a decrease in the proportion of children who brush their teeth twice a day with fluoridated toothpaste (many children only brush once a day) and the consumption of soft drinks, cordial and juices rather than fluoridated tap water. This reinforces the point that any gains achieved in oral health within a community can be rapidly lost if there are changes in dietary practices and oral health care.

Given that there are twenty primary teeth and that the sizes of these teeth are correlated — that is, if a central incisor is larger than average in a child, then the other teeth will also tend to be larger — it was clear that statistical approaches would be needed to analyse our data that could take account of intercorrelations between variables. These types of analyses which include many intercorrelated variables are referred to as multivariate analyses. It was particularly important for the proposed multivariate studies that full sets of data were obtained for as many children as possible, because missing values always pose a problem for such analyses. As very few children in the 4-6-year-old age group were likely to have received any orthodontic treatment, the problems of selection bias that can be a major confounding problem for studies of the permanent dentition were also overcome to a large extent.

Following discussions with the NHMRC Twin Registry, from whom it was intended to recruit twins for the study, it was clear that a large proportion of the twins enrolled with the Registry were in the 2-6-year-old age bracket. This provided an excellent pool of potential participants. We had also estimated that there were around 200 pairs of twins, enrolled with the Registry, who fell within the desired age group and were living in the Adelaide metropolitan area.

Reflecting on the Foreword written by Nick Martin and colleagues to the papers arising from the 12th International Congress on Twin Studies in Belgium, published in the journal *Behavior Genetics* (Martin et al., 1989; see also page 13 of Chapter Four), we were aware that many of the previous twin studies of dental morphology had employed rather simplistic analyses and focused almost entirely on trying to estimate heritabilities.

Around this time, the methods of genetic analysis of covariance structure that had been introduced by Karl Jöreskog in the early 1970s (Jöreskog, 1973), which had then been adapted by Nick Martin and Lyndon Eaves (Martin and Eaves, 1977), were being further developed. For example, Andrew Heath and colleagues, and Mike Neale and Lon Cardon were developing powerful new methods that would enable hypotheses about the structure of variation within, as well as covariation between, variables to be tested.

In the 1990s, Professor Mike Neale from the Medical College of Virginia, USA, the author of LISREL and Mx manuals for genetic modelling, visited Adelaide and provided us with very helpful advice about how to apply his software to our dental data. Although opportunities for face-to-face contact have been limited since then, Professor Neale has provided our group, especially Paula Dempsey throughout her PhD (Dempsey et al., 1995) and more recently Associate Professor Toby Hughes, with invaluable advice, and we are very grateful that he continues to do so. Some of the advantages of using LISREL and its successor, Mx, are that they allow various genetic models to be fitted to the data that have been collected, and then these models can be tested statistically to assess their goodness-of-fit to the data.

It was decided to use the software program Mx, developed by Mike Neale, to analyse our dental data from Australian twins. A collaboration had already been commenced with Nick Martin applying Mx to dental crown measurements of the permanent dentitions of teenage twins (Cohort 1), but it was now planned to extend these studies to include the primary dentition (Cohort 2), and eventually to analyse data from both dentitions of individuals to see whether the same genetic factors operated over time, influencing the development of both sets of teeth.

Mx is essentially an improved version of LISREL, the linear structural modelling program that was developed by Karl Jöreskog and Dag Sörbom (1989). The advantage of Mx over previous approaches for analysing twin data was that it enabled various genetic models to be fitted to correlation matrices by a method referred to as maximum likelihood. Initially, the pre-processing package PRELIS was used to generate the correlation matrices from raw data for monozygotic and dizygotic twin pairs. Different models could then be tested using Chi-square tests to determine the goodness-of-fit of the data to the models; and then estimates of the model parameters — for example, additive genetic variance and environmental variance, as well as their standard errors — could be obtained.

This innovation represented a major advance over traditional methods, which were based on various assumptions and did not provide for different models to be tested, one after the other, to see how well they fitted the data. Previous methods tended to lead to the calculation of estimates of heritability based on simple formulae, and did not enable standard errors of estimates to be calculated readily. The use of LISREL and Mx was facilitated by the application of path analysis, which enabled path diagrams to be generated. (For an example of a path diagram, see Figure 5.1 below.) These diagrams showed the relationships of the so-called latent (or hidden) variables which represented genetic and environmental causes of individual differences to the dental and facial features being measured — that is, the various dento-facial phenotypes. Mx also provided a number of particularly useful additional features, including the ability to model group means and to test for sex-limitation and interactions between the genotype and environment.

Cohort 2 – A longitudinal study of dental and facial development

Figure 5.1 presents a simple path diagram of a structural equation model (SEM) representing the twin relationship for a single trait. Variation in the observed twin phenotypes (square boxes) is influenced by a number of latent (unmeasured) variables (circles). Broadly speaking, these are the additive effects of an individual's genes (A), the non-additive effects (dominance, epistasis) of an individual's genes (D), the influence of the environment shared by co-twins (C), and the unique environment experienced by an individual twin (E). This last variable also encapsulates experimental error. The model completely decomposes observed variation into a number of discrete linear relationships between latent and measured variables, related by a series of parameters (a, d, c and e) which can be estimated using likelihood-based approaches. The 'structural' elements of the model (intra-pair correlations, r) capitalise on the observer's knowledge of biology underpinning the relationships between latent variables. To this end, additive genetic effects have a correlation (r) of 1.0 in monozygotic twins, and 0.5 in dizygotic twins. Unsurprisingly, the correlation between shared environments is 1.0 regardless of zygosity for twins raised together.

It was also decided to use the co-twin control design where appropriate. As we explained in Chapter Three, this model involves studying pairs of monozygotic twins where one member of the pair may have been exposed to a different treatment

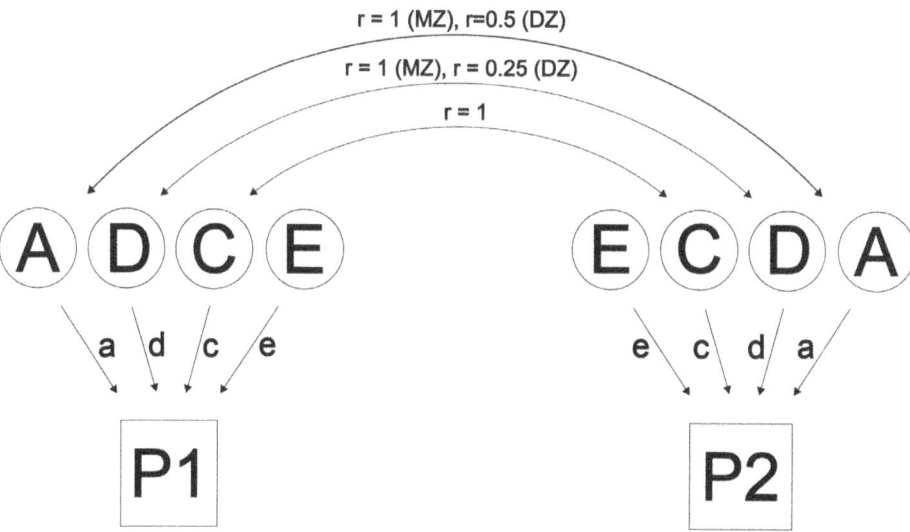

Figure 5.1
Path diagram showing the relationships between a pair of twins for a single trait.

or experience than the other. Assuming that all other influential environmental factors are the same in each twin, the differences observed between monozygotic co-twins can be related to the treatment or the different experience. It was felt that this design would be relevant to comparisons of various dental and facial features. For example, it would be possible to look at differences in expression of various dental anomalies between monozygotic co-twins, such as congenitally missing teeth or extra (supernumerary) teeth. There was also the possibility of exploring the outcomes when one twin displayed a habit, such as thumb-sucking, and the other did not; or where one co-twin had orthodontic treatment and the other did not. At that time, there was very little literature published on what role epigenetic factors might play as a source of differences between monozygotic co-twins.

COLLECTION OF RECORDS AND EXAMINATION OF TWINS

Twins were recruited from the NHMRC Twin Registry in Melbourne and invitations to participate were mailed to twin families in Adelaide and Melbourne. Professor Louise Brearley Messer, a specialist paediatric dentist at the Dental School in Melbourne, was contacted, and she agreed to join the study (Figure 5.2).

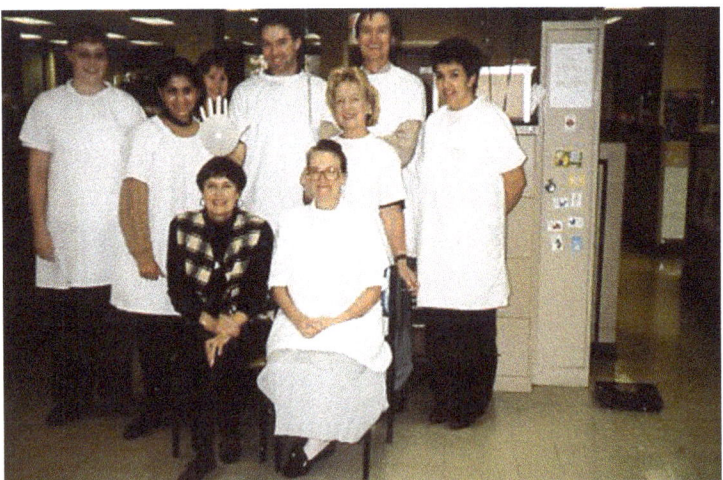

Figure 5.2
Sandy Pinkerton (front left) with Professor Louise Brearley Messer (front right) with other members of the Melbourne team.

Cohort 2 – A longitudinal study of dental and facial development

The initial plan was to examine and obtain records of around 250 pairs of twins in Adelaide and Melbourne in the 4-6-year-old age bracket. It was envisaged that about fifty pairs of twins would be recruited into each of the following five groups: monozygotic twin boys, monozygotic twin girls, dizygotic twin boys, dizygotic twin girls, dizygotic boy/girl pairs.

It was planned to obtain a comprehensive range of observations and records from the twins, including direct examinations of their teeth and oral structures, to record teeth present, dental caries, restorations, dental anomalies (such as missing teeth, fused teeth, extra teeth), and type of occlusion. It was also important to arrange for the necessary photographic equipment and other items to be ready at each appointment in the Adelaide and Melbourne Dental Hospitals. Logistical demands were made even more difficult, as it was intended to obtain fingerprints and dental impressions using alginate impression material from which study models would be poured up in dental stone. Stone dental models have the advantage of providing permanent records of the dentitions of twins which can be studied for years and years — the only disadvantage being the space they take for storage. Recently, orthodontists have begun producing 'virtual models', which are produced by obtaining 3D scans of impressions or previously obtained dental models. This is clearly a development with important research implications, provided the accuracy of the virtual models can be shown to be good enough. We are in the process of scanning all of our dental models, not only as a means of saving space but also as a back-up for the original models in case they are damaged.

Initially, it was unclear how difficult it would be to obtain high-quality dental impressions from children who would be only 4 to 6 years of age. Although several members of the research team who had been assembled were dentists, managing young children in the dental surgery can be tricky, and there was some concern that specialist input from a paediatric dentist might be needed to ensure that the impressions were of high enough quality to enable the acquisition of highly precise measurements. Our plan was to examine primary teeth of the twins soon after they were all present in the mouth (usually by around 4 years of age) and then again when the twins were around 9 to 11 years old (when there is usually a mix of primary and permanent teeth), and then a third time when they were 12 to 14 years old (when all of the permanent teeth have usually emerged except for the third molars).

The length of time this longitudinal project would involve was also a matter for some concern initially. Would the study be able to hold the interest of the children over those years? Would the families be available for the arranged appointments? To cover the second problem, concerning appointment availability, twin appointments were made when school holidays and the university vacations overlapped, so that parents, twins, their siblings, postgraduate dentists and academic staff could be available at the same time. Importantly, too, would it be possible to obtain the continual funding required to run a longitudinal study?

As it turned out, the clinical procedures went well, with good dental impressions being obtained from most of the children, even the 4- and 5-year-olds, and the interest of both parents and children remained excellent (Figure 5.3). To many of the researchers it was a revelation that the parents responded so well to the requirements of the study, with many parents freely giving their time and covering their own expenses to travel large distances to attend the clinical sessions. After the first field trip to Melbourne in July 1995, another trip was arranged in September of the same year. Then a return trip was made in January 1996. The combined collection of records obtained in both

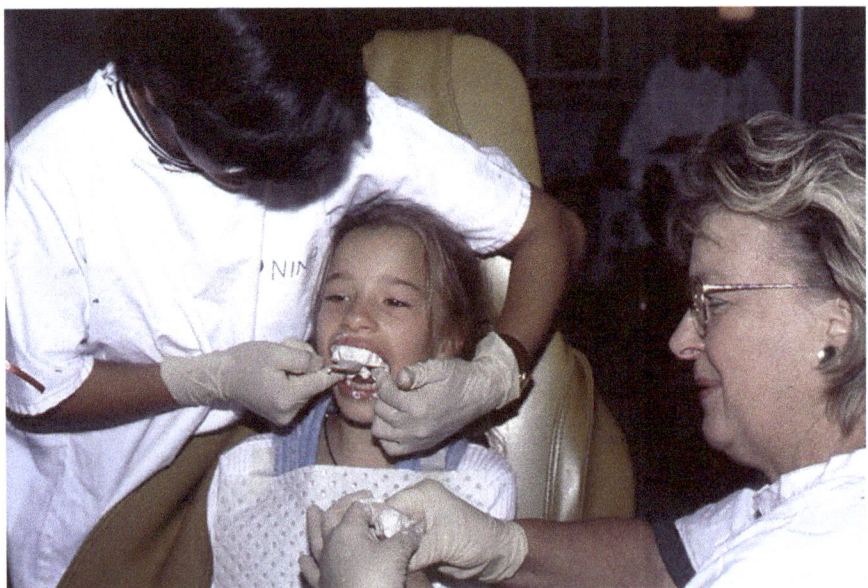

Figure 5.3
Dental assistant modelling a ghost on a twin's finger whilst her impression was being obtained by a dentist. Melbourne session, September 1998.

Cohort 2 – A longitudinal study of dental and facial development

Adelaide and Melbourne for those six months totalled 200 twin pairs (Figure 5.4). One of the most important issues to consider when making alginate impressions is the ability to pour dental stone into the impressions as soon as possible. Therefore, in both Melbourne and Adelaide, it was essential to be able to have a fast and reliable service to pour the impressions in stone before the impression material became distorted. This was achieved by having dedicated laboratory technicians or senior dental students on hand throughout the period of the visits.

Another important requirement in the acquisition of records was the need to obtain fingerprints from the young participants. Grant Townsend had commenced collecting fingerprints and palm-prints (dermatoglyphics) of twins and family members during the data collection in Cohort 1 (see Chapter Four). The children particularly enjoyed getting their fingers dirty with printer's ink when making

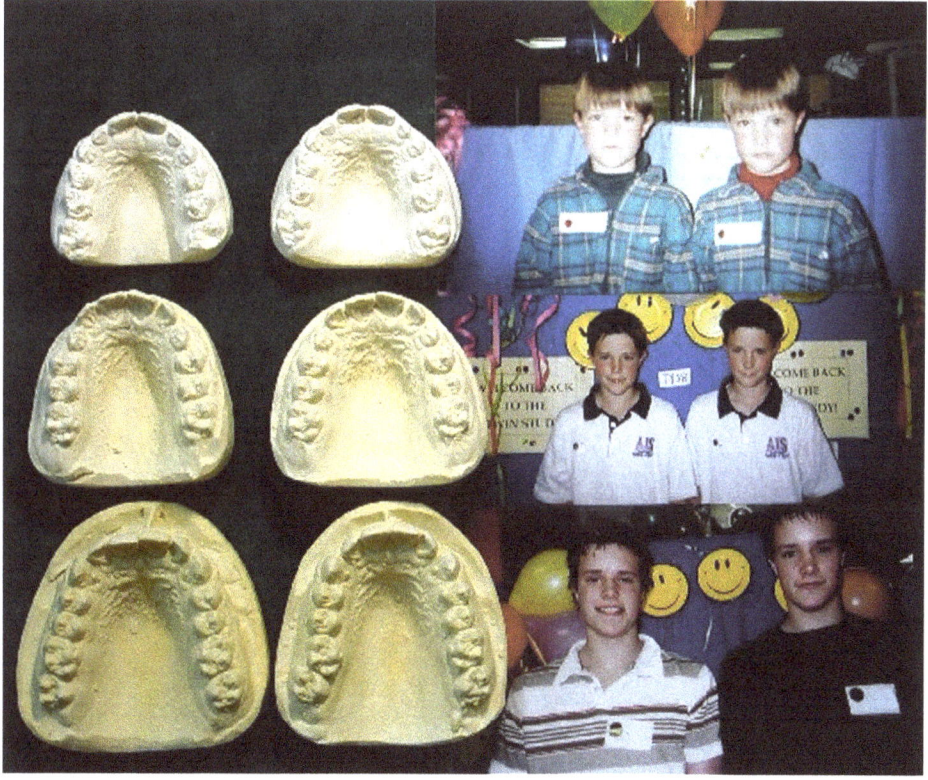

Figure 5.4
Serial upper dental models of a pair of twins in Cohort 2.

fingerprints. These records added to those already acquired, which we hope will establish whether there are common genetic factors that influence the size, shape and patterning of teeth and fingerprints within individuals (Figure 5.5).

Hand, eye and foot preference records were also collected. Based upon the Edinburgh Inventory (Oldfield, 1971), testing was conducted for hand, eye and foot dominance. Previously, with the teenage twins in Cohort 1, a small number of items had been used to remind the twins whether they predominantly used their left or right hand when carrying out a task. With much younger participants in Cohort 2, an 'obstacle course' was devised, designed to downplay the fact that this was a test and to replace it with entertaining tasks. Balls were kicked and thrown around, and toy telescopes and microscopes were used. The children had fun (and so did we) as their hand, eye and foot actions were noted. It was easier, and more objective, to observe them at play with their unconscious actions than it was to ask them direct questions. Parental comments after watching their children play were important in order to

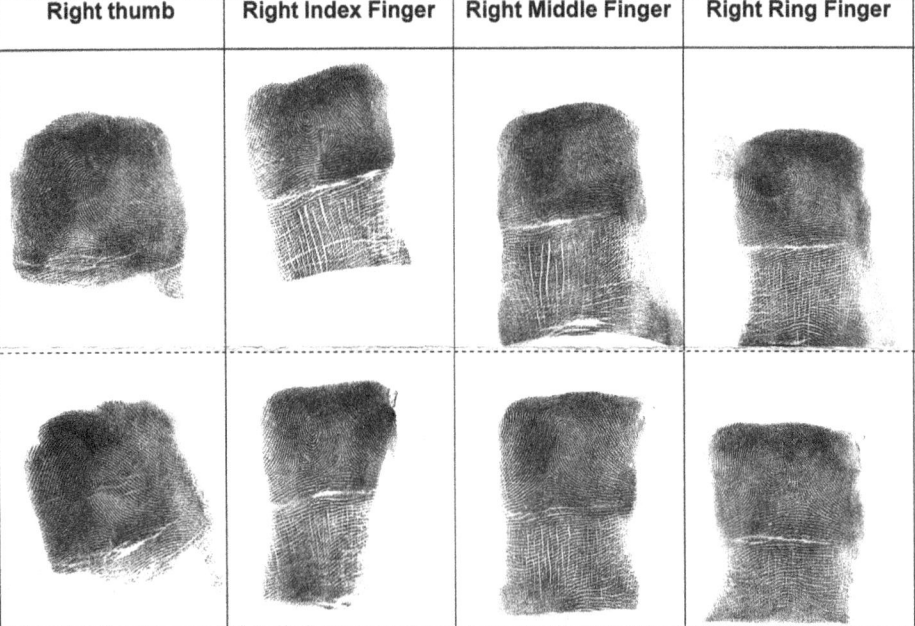

Figure 5.5
Comparison of fingerprint patterns in a pair of monozygotic twins (above and below). The patterns are very similar but not identical.

Cohort 2 – A longitudinal study of dental and facial development

compare what was observed at home and what the researchers observed during the testing period.

It was decided that it would be valuable to ask the parents of the twins to gather their twins' primary (baby) teeth as they were lost (or shed). Sophisticated imaging techniques were becoming available and, although they were still very expensive at that time, it was thought that the teeth could be kept in storage until it became feasible to scan them later on. This would enable the different dental tissues composing teeth to be examined in detail — for example, the enamel, dentine and pulp cavities.

Previous research with Professor Lassi Alvesalo and his colleagues in Finland had been aimed at clarifying the roles of the sex chromosomes in human dental development. By measuring tooth crowns on intra-oral radiographs obtained from individuals with extra or missing sex chromosomes, it was evident that the thickness of the enamel and dentine varied significantly as the number of X and Y chromosomes varied. In fact, the X chromosome appeared to mainly regulate enamel thickness, with increasing thickness being associated with more X chromosomes. In contrast, the Y chromosome seemed to affect both enamel and dentine thickness (Alvesalo et al., 2009; 2013). Using exfoliated teeth from the twins, it is now planned to further explore the roles of genetic and environmental influences on the dental tissues, to build on the pioneering work of Lassi Alvesalo and his team.

Meanwhile, it was decided that during the visits to Melbourne we would continue to obtain facial photographs in a standardised manner, as had been done for Cohort 1. This was one aspect of the study where Louise Messer's expertise and access

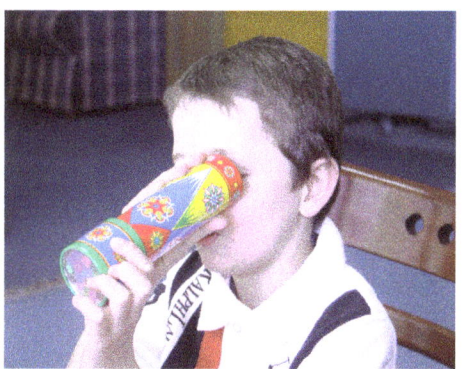 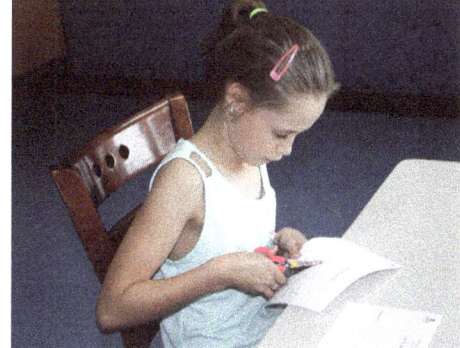

Figure 5.6
Testing eye dominance and hand dominance.

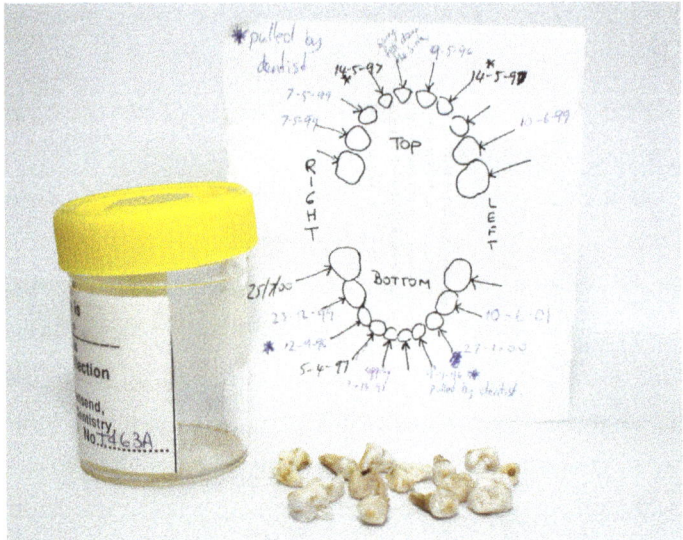

Figure 5.7
Exfoliated primary teeth with chart recording the dates when teeth were shed.

to a standardised 2D photographic system in Melbourne proved to be invaluable, and the equipment that was used is described in more detail later in this chapter. Medical histories of the mothers during pregnancy were also recorded, including placenta type (for example, whether one or two placentas were present), and also information about smoking and alcohol consumption.

Cohort 2 as a longitudinal study

There are definite advantages in carrying out longitudinal growth studies of humans rather than using the more common cross-sectional approach. Given that we all grow and develop at different times and rates, the best way to accurately characterise the growth process is to follow individuals throughout their period of growth, rather than to group children of different ages together and examine them only once. However, by their very nature, longitudinal studies take a long time to complete, so there is inevitably attrition of participants over time, as they move to other places or lose interest in the study. There is also the issue of ongoing commitment by the researchers and, of course, the high cost involved. We knew that we were committed enough to ensure that we would maintain our enthusiasm for the proposed research, but the funding of these types of studies is always problematic. For longitudinal studies, it is essential to have ongoing funding, and we were acutely aware when we commenced this study that we would be reliant on continual funding from the NHMRC and other funding bodies.

In terms of the potential significance of the proposed research, it was very apparent to us that a better understanding was needed of how genetic and environmental factors influenced dental and facial growth over time in young, growing children. This would provide a stronger scientific basis for early preventive and treatment-planning approaches in those individuals who develop disharmonies of the teeth and/or jaws, such as crooked teeth or altered contact between the dental arches. These disharmonies are commonly described as 'malocclusions', but they actually represent the extremes of normal variation in the development of the dentition. Furthermore, there is no definite 'cut-off point' beyond which it can be stated definitively that a malocclusion is present or not. Thus it is imperative to understand how genetic and environmental factors, and also epigenetic factors, influence normal growth and development before we can hope to understand the factors that contribute to the variation observed in the number, size, shape and arrangement of teeth in the population at large.

Dental malocclusion represents a significant problem in Australia, with the prevalence estimated to be around 60 per cent, and treatment costs running into millions of dollars per year. More recently, there has been increased interest in early intervention to prevent malocclusions, but relatively little is known about the appropriate age at which to intervene, or about the effectiveness of early treatment in the longer term.

Around the time that we were beginning our longitudinal study, Juha Varrela and Pentti Alanen (1995) made the following statement in an editorial in the top-ranking dental research journal, the *Journal of Dental Research*: 'There is a clear need for research programs on early occlusal and craniofacial development from the point of view of prevention and early treatment'. Juha Varrela is Professor of Orthodontics at the University of Turku in Finland, and for many years he has been a pioneer in treating occlusal problems in the primary dentition phase, so it was very encouraging to read this statement. We felt we were on the right track!

Given the early timing of development of the primary teeth, it was also thought that this study should help to better understand the early developmental events in the twinning process, including the determination of body symmetry and the phenomenon of mirror imaging.

As the plans for running an ongoing longitudinal study of dental and facial growth and morphology developed further, we realised that we would need to 'package' the study into components when seeking support for funding from the NHMRC. After successfully collecting records of over 300 pairs of twins at the primary dentition phase, we felt confident that we could extend the study to include re-examining the same twins at two other important milestones in terms of their dental development — at the mixed dentition stage around 8 to 10 years of age, and then again at the permanent dentition phase, around 12 to 14 years of age. It was decided to concentrate initially on the collection of records and acquisition of data at the mixed dentition stage, while simultaneously testing several hypotheses relating to the primary and mixed dentitions. Fortunately, this proved to be a successful strategy and we received funding from the NHMRC which enabled us to move forward with the study. We realised that we would need to travel to Melbourne to examine many of the twins, so we were very pleased to extend our ongoing collaboration with Louise Messer, who was a Chief Investigator on our NHMRC grant application.

Twins in Melbourne

As the study proceeded, the exploration of facial morphology became centred on the Dental School in Melbourne, where an orthogonal photographic system had been set up in the Department of Orthodontics. Professor Louise Brearley Messer took charge of photographing the twins when they came to the School for their dental appointments. The system allowed a right facial profile and a frontal view to be obtained simultaneously under standardised conditions of lighting and facial position. The frontal images could be used for linear and plane measurements, and the profiles could be used for Fourier analysis. We had also developed software to allow us to calculate the 3D co-ordinates of facial reference points, taking into account scaling factors and the geometry.

It was decided to record some additional features of the dentition, as well as those already mentioned. These included wear facets on teeth, which indicated the nature and extent of tooth wear that had occurred. Wear facets on opposing teeth that can only be matched in extreme, eccentric jaw positions provide evidence that individuals have been grinding their teeth. The term often used to describe this

Cohort 2 – A longitudinal study of dental and facial development

activity is 'bruxism' and this is an activity that commonly occurs at night while we are asleep. The aetiology of bruxism remains a contentious area in dentistry, with some researchers emphasising the importance of local factors within the dentition (for example, occlusal interferences between opposing teeth), and others favouring an origin within the central nervous system, linked to stress. Our twin data provided an ideal opportunity to try to unravel the relative importance of genetic and environmental influences on wear facet frequency and patterning, and hence to clarify what the underlying causes of tooth grinding might be.

We also decided to examine the teeth of the twins for evidence of enamel hypoplasia. This condition includes a variety of quantitative developmental defects that may be evident on dental crowns as single or multiple pits, small furrows, deep and wide troughs, or entirely missing enamel. Hypoplasias evident in fully formed teeth result from disruptions of enamel formation which are thought to reflect compromised nutritional status or developmental insults at the time of crown formation. Although the position of a hypoplastic defect on the crown of a tooth enables the timing of the insult to be inferred, the relative roles of genetic and environmental factors in determining the expression of these defects is still unclear (refer to Figure 1.20 in Chapter One). The detailed medical histories that we were

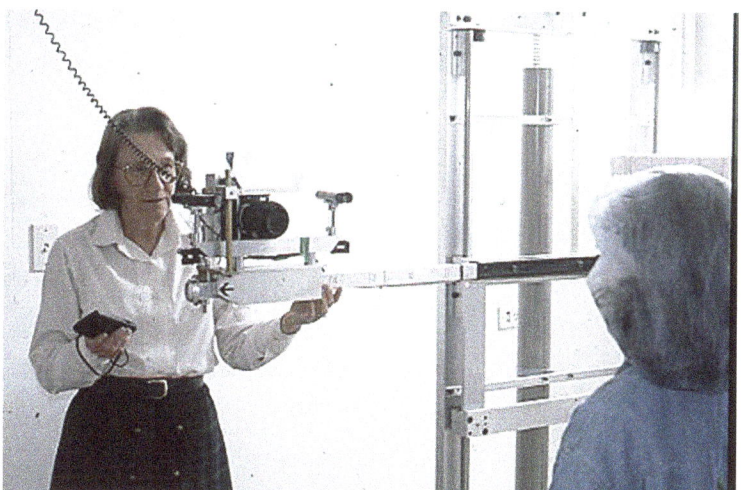

Figure 5.8
Professor Louise Brearley Messer obtaining standardised facial photographs of a twin enrolled in Cohort 2.

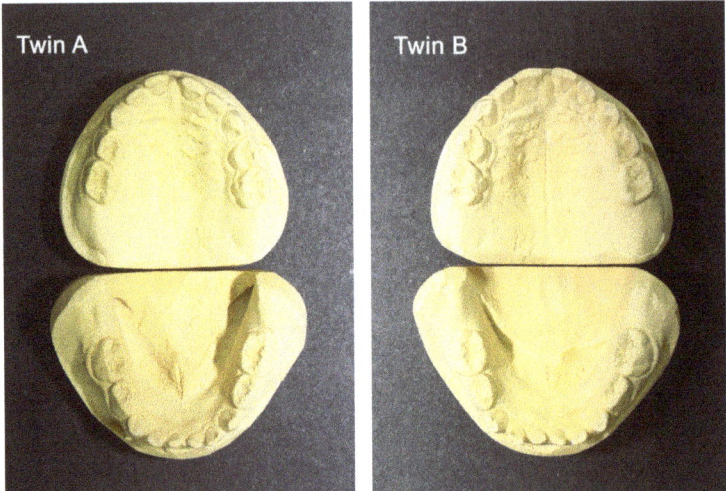

Figure 5.9
Dental models of a pair of monozygotic twins showing similar patterns of tooth wear.

collecting on maternal health and postnatal development of the twins enabled us to explore associations between developmental disturbances and expression of hypoplastic defects.

As so often happens in longitudinal studies, fresh ideas are generated and new initiatives developed during the course of an ongoing research project. As our understanding of the role of genetic influences on variation in dento-facial features improved, we became increasingly interested in the relationships between tooth emergence and initial colonisation of bacteria in the mouth. There was evidence that those individuals who became colonised with *Streptococcus mutans* at an earlier age were more likely to suffer from dental decay subsequently. Thus it seemed to us that studying the roles of genetic and environmental factors on the formation and composition of dental plaque in twins offered great promise for the eventual development of new, biologically based, preventive methods to protect against the development of dental decay. These ideas stimulated us to decide to commence a third major study of twins and their families, now referred to as Cohort 3. We will discuss Cohort 3 further in the following chapter.

Cohort 2 – A longitudinal study of dental and facial development

SOME KEY FINDINGS OF OUR STUDIES INVOLVING COHORT 2

1. One of our first studies of the primary dentition of twins involved recording the prevalence of spacing between the teeth of children between the ages of 4 to 7 years. Our studies showed that spacing was present in the primary dentition in most of the children examined (so it can be considered a 'normal' feature at these ages), and that there was a genetic basis to the observed variation (Thomas and Townsend, 1999).

2. Fluctuating dental asymmetry (FDA) refers to the small, random differences in size between corresponding teeth on opposite sides of the dental arch. Increased levels of FDA have been reported in individuals with congenital abnormalities and genetic syndromes. Associations have also been noted with inbreeding and various environmental factors, such as noise, temperature, and maternal smoking and alcohol consumption. Interestingly, this study showed evidence of significant FDA in the sample of twins studied, but there was also some evidence of directional dental asymmetry, with some teeth being consistently larger on one side than the other. This is a feature that continues to perplex researchers and is currently under investigation. Our study failed to confirm the assertion of Boklage that twins are more symmetrical in their dental dimensions than singletons; but ours was only based on univariate analyses, rather than the multivariate analysis undertaken by Boklage (Townsend et al., 1999).

3. As our sample of twins at the mixed dentition stage of development grew, it became possible to study the expression of different dental features in the primary and permanent dentitions of the same individuals — for example, Carabelli trait. This is a major advantage of studying the teeth of children in the mixed dentition phase of development, as the primary molars and the permanent first molar are present in the mouth at the same time. Thus this offers a 'longitudinal view' of dental development in a single 'snapshot' of time. Our studies confirmed that similar genetic factors are likely to be involved in influencing the expression of Carabelli trait on the upper molar teeth, but that the contribution of environmental factors is likely to be more evident in the permanent first molar, which develops over a longer period of time, than in the primary second molar,

which completes its crown development by around twelve months postnatally (Pinkerton et al., 1999).

4. One study that took advantage of the differences in birth dates of the twins comprising Cohort 1 and those in Cohort 2 was a study of enamel hypoplasia undertaken with Professor Rob Corruccini from the USA. Enamel hypoplasias represent disruptions in the calcification process during enamel formation, which are considered to reflect a response to metabolic stress during the period of dental crown development. A notable reduction in the frequency of hypoplasias was noted between those twins born around 1965 (Cohort 1) and those born around 1990 (Cohort 2). While a reduction in childhood fevers and clinical intervention to reduce stresses around birth may have contributed to these findings, the strongest hypoplasia-preventing factor appeared to be the introduction of water fluoridation into the water supply (Corruccini and Townsend, 2003).

5. Another study looked at the prevalence of tooth grinding in young twins, based on the presence of wear facets on the tips of the canine teeth. Evidence of tooth grinding was found in all of the twins studied, and it was often expressed more on one side than the other. There was also some evidence of a mirror imaging effect for tooth grinding in some of the monozygotic twin pairs (Dooland et al., 2006).

6. A series of papers with Toby Hughes as the first author provided a much clearer picture of the role of genetic factors on observed variation in the primary dentition than was available previously. This was due to the application of modern methods of genetic model-fitting and the availability of relatively large sample sizes. These findings have important implications for dental anthropologists and clinicians (Hughes et al., 2000; Hughes et al., 2001).

7. A study of the associations between birthweight and tooth size in twins in Cohort 2 showed some evidence for a reduction in tooth size in the female twins who were of low birthweight, but there was no evidence of any reduction in the males. The reduction was small in magnitude, being only 2 to 3 per cent in both the primary and the permanent incisor teeth. These findings confirmed the general view that the developing

teeth are well protected from developmental disturbances during pre- and postnatal periods (Apps et al., 2004).

8. Chorion type (that is, whether one or two placentas are present when twins are born) is an important factor to remember when considering the development of monozygotic twins, as vascular anastomoses (connections) between monochorionic monozygotic twins can lead to an imbalance in development between co-twins. In a study carried out by an Honours student, Jonathan Race, it was found that maternal reports were unreliable for determining chorion type, and hospital records often did not provide enough information to be certain about chorionicity. Large birthweight differences were found to occur more often in monochorionic twins pairs than dichorionic pairs in the study sample (Race et al., 2006). Greater emphasis is now being placed on accurate diagnosis of chorion type in twin studies, as it is appreciated that not all monozygotic twins should be lumped together for analysis. If we were commencing another twin study now, we would certainly aim to include accurate information on chorion type, and this has been made more feasible by the developments in ultrasonography that enable chorion type to be determined non-invasively at around eleven to fourteen weeks in utero.

9. The aim of a study reported in the *Australian Dental Journal* in 2005 (Townsend et al., 2005) was to determine the prevalence of discordant expression (that is, differences in expression) for missing teeth and extra teeth in a sample of 278 monozygotic twin pairs, and to explain how the differences in appearance (phenotypic differences) may have occurred despite the similar genotypes of co-twins. At least one missing upper lateral incisor or second premolar was noted in 24 of the 278 twin pairs (8.6 per cent), with 21 of these 24 pairs (87.5 per cent) showing discordant expression. Nine of the 278 twin pairs had extra teeth (supernumeraries), with 8 of the 9 pairs (88.9 per cent) being discordant. These findings showed that differences in expression of missing or extra teeth are common in monozygotic twin pairs, even though their genetic codes are identical. We suggested that minor variations in epigenetic events during tooth formation (that is, the way in which their genes are expressed) may lead to quite distinct differences in their dental phenotypes (the number of teeth

present). This was one of the first papers to raise the issue of epigenetic influences on dental development based on studies of monozygotic twins.

10. A paper in the *Journal of Dental Research*, based on the PhD studies of Daniela Ribeiro, was the first to investigate both primary and permanent tooth sizes in females from opposite-sex dizygotic twin pairs compared with females from dizygotic same-sex and monozygotic twin pairs to indicate the intra-uterine influence of male hormones on dental development. This paper built on the earlier work of Paula Dempsey, which concentrated on the permanent dentition only (Dempsey et al., 1995). The findings of Ribeiro's study provide strong support for the Twin Testosterone Transfer (TTT) hypothesis, and we have proposed that, together, the effects of sex hormones and intra-uterine male hormone levels influence different tooth dimensions and contribute differentially to sexual dimorphism in the size of human teeth (Ribeiro et al., 2013).

References

Alvesalo L (2009). Human sex chromosomes in oral and craniofacial growth. *Arch Oral Biol* 54S:S18-S24.

Alvesalo L (2013). The expression of human sex chromosome genes in oral and craniofacial growth. In: *Anthropological Perspectives on Tooth Morphology: genetics, evolution, variation.* Scott GR, Irish JD, editors. Cambridge: Cambridge University Press, pp. 92-107.

Apps MV, Hughes TE, Townsend GC (2004). The effect of birthweight on tooth size variability in twins. *Twin Res* 7:415-420.

Corruccini RS, Townsend GC (2003). Decline in enamel hypoplasia in relation to fluoridation in Australians. *Am J Hum Biol* 15:795-799.

Dempsey PJ, Townsend GC, Martin NG, Neale MC (1995). Genetic covariance structure of incisor crown size in twins. *J Dent Res* 74:1389-1398.

Dooland KV, Townsend GC, Kaidonis JA (2006). Prevalence and side preference for tooth grinding in twins. *Aust Dent J* 51:219-224.

Ha D, Roberts-Thomson K, Armfield J (2011). The Child Dental Health Surveys Australia, 2005 and 2006. *Dental statistics and research series no. 54. Cat. no. DEN 213.* Canberra: Australian Institute of Health and Welfare. http://www.aihw.gov.au/publication-detail/?id=10737420637. Accessed 21 May 2015.

Hughes T, Dempsey P, Richards L, Townsend G (2000). Genetic analysis of deciduous tooth size in Australian twins. *Arch Oral Biol* 45:997-1004.

Hughes T, Thomas C, Townsend G (2001). A study of occlusal variation in the primary dentition of Australian twins and singletons. *Arch Oral Biol* 46:857-864.

Jöreskog KG (1973). Analysis of covariance structures. In: *Multivariate Analysis-III Proceedings of the Third International Symposium on Multivariate Analysis held at Wright State University, Dayton, Ohio, June 19–24.* Krishnaiah PR, editor. New York: Academic Press, pp. 263-285.

Jöreskog KG, Sörbom D (1989). *LISREL 7 user's reference guide.* Chicago: Scientific Software Inc.

Martin NG, Boomsma DI, Neale MC (1989). Foreword. *Behav Genet* 19:5-7.

Martin NG, Eaves LJ (1977). The genetic analysis of covariance structure. *Heredity* 38:79-95.

Oldfield RC (1971). The assessment and analysis of handedness: the Edinburgh Inventory. *Neuropsychologia* 9:97-113.

Pinkerton S, Townsend G, Richards L, Schwerdt W, Dempsey P (1999). Expression of Carabelli trait in both dentitions of Australian twins. *Perspec Hum Biol* 4(3):19-28.

Race JP, Townsend GC, Hughes TE (2006). Chorion type, birth weight discordance and tooth-size variability in Australian monozygotic twins. *Twin Res Hum Genet* 9:285-291.

Ribeiro DC, Brook AH, Hughes TE, Sampson WJ, Townsend GC (2013). Intrauterine hormone effects on tooth dimensions. *J Dent Res* 92:425-431.

Thomas CJ, Townsend GC (1999). Anterior spacing in the primary dentition: a study of Australian twins and singletons. *Perspec Hum Biol* 4(3):29-35.

Townsend G, Dempsey P, Richards L (1999). Asymmetry in the deciduous dentition: fluctuating and directional components. *Perspec Hum Biol* 4(3):45-52.

Townsend GC, Richards L, Hughes T, Pinkerton S, Schwerdt W (2005). Epigenetic influences may explain dental differences in monozygotic twin pairs. *Aust Dent J* 50:95-100.

Varrela J, Alanen P (1995). Prevention and early treatment in orthodontics: a perspective. *J Dent Res* 74:1436-1438.

Chapter Six

COHORT 3 – TOOTH EMERGENCE AND ORAL HEALTH IN AUSTRALIAN TWINS AND THEIR FAMILIES

Introduction

While the focus of our studies involving Cohorts 1 and 2 was on dental development and morphology, we decided to concentrate more on oral health and disease, particularly dental decay, when studying Cohort 3. The major developments in molecular biology have also enabled research involving this cohort to make use of new technologies and approaches to study genetic effects more directly.

Dental decay (caries) is the most common chronic disease affecting Australian children, despite the implementation of public health initiatives, such as fluoridated drinking water and toothpastes. The disease can cause pain and systemic infection, lead to speech and learning problems, and is a predictor for poor general health. Treatment for dental caries inflicts a huge economic burden on society, accounting for 6.5 per cent ($AUS5.3 billion) of total health care expenditure in Australia per year (Armfield et al., 2009; Ha et al., 2011).

In 2004, we submitted an application for funding to the NHMRC for a new initiative involving Australian twins and their families. The title of this grant application was 'Tooth emergence and oral streptococci colonisation: a longitudinal study of Australian twins'. Although the application was supported, funding was only provided for three years rather than the five years that had been requested. The study commenced in 2005, with the twins and their families comprising what is now referred to as Cohort 3. The chief investigators on this project were Grant Townsend, Kim Seow, Theo Gotjamanos, Toby Hughes, Neville Gully and Lindsay Richards.

The first aim of the project was to clarify the influences of genetic and environmental determinants on variation in the emergence (often referred to as tooth eruption) of the human primary teeth by applying modern methods of genetic model-fitting to longitudinal data obtained from young monozygotic and dizygotic twin pairs. The intention was to compare variability in both the timing and sequencing of tooth emergence within and between the twins, and to relate these findings to measures of physical development and other pre- and postnatal factors. It was also planned to apply linkage analyses to detect quantitative trait loci (QTLs) for dental development using genome scans of DNA derived from cheek cells.

QTLs refer to regions of the DNA which contain, or are linked to, genes that influence a particular quantitative feature or trait. By statistically linking phenotypic data (obtained through the analysis of trait measurements) and genotypic data (acquired through the use of identifying molecular markers), it is possible to explain the genetic basis of variation in complex traits, such as dental caries (Miles and Wayne, 2008).

The second aim of the project was to study the relationship between the timing of emergence of the primary teeth and the colonisation of the oral cavity by mutans streptococci, bacteria known to be important in the development of dental decay (dental caries). It was also planned, subject to ongoing funding, to examine the twins as they grew older to record the development of any dental decay or the presence of developmental enamel defects.

In order to better understand how genetic factors contribute to dental caries, it was decided to determine the degree to which genetic and environmental factors influence microbial species associated with decay and oral health. Using the traditional twin model method, comparisons of monozygotic and dizygotic twin pairs would be used to investigate the role of genetic factors, as well as shared and non-shared environmental factors, in contributing to phenotypic variation. This model relies on the fact that monozygotic twins have identical genotypes, whereas dizygotic twins share on average half their genes. It is usually assumed that for twins who are living together, the effect of shared environment on both monozygotic and dizygotic twins will be equivalent. Hence, any feature that shows greater associations between pairs of monozygotic twins compared with dizygotic twins indicates the influence of genetic factors.

Cohort 3 – Tooth emergence and oral health in Australian twins

Professor Kim Seow and her team of researchers from Queensland had established the timing of initial colonisation of mutans streptococci in the mouths of pre-term and full-term children from birth to 24 months of age (Wan et al., 2001a,b; 2003). These studies had shown that mutans streptococci colonisation steadily increases with increasing age and number of teeth. They had also identified important infant and maternal factors associated with the acquisition of mutans streptococci. So we were very interested in seeing what sort of relationships might occur in monozygotic and dizygotic twins in relation to colonisation, tooth emergence and oral health. Was there evidence that genetic factors played an important role in these processes?

Another of our collaborators, Professor Theo Gotjamanos from the Fremantle campus of the University of Notre Dame Australia, had noted that the primary teeth of Australian children seemed to be erupting later than expected according to published standards. A similar trend had also been reported for the permanent teeth in Australian children (Diamanti and Townsend, 2003). Professor Gotjamanos had suggested that delayed timing of emergence of the primary teeth might be a contributory factor in an observed decline of dental caries affecting the primary teeth of Australian children at that time. This altered 'window of infectivity', as it had been

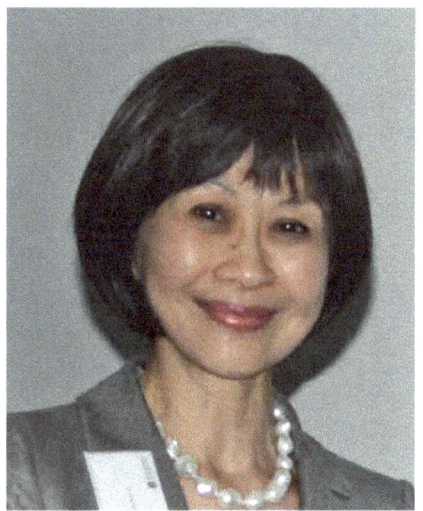

Figure 6.1
Professor Kim Seow, University of Queensland.

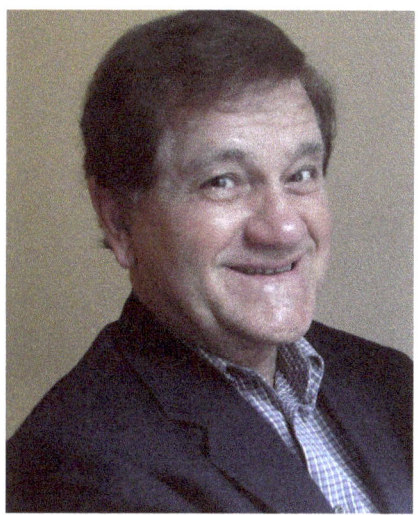

Figure 6.2
Professor Theo Gotjamanos, University of Notre Dame Western Australia.

termed by Page Caufield and colleagues (1993), was thought to be characterised by delayed colonisation by mutans streptococci on newly emerged teeth.

Published literature at the time also suggested that children infected with mutans streptococci before the age of 3 years had a greater prevalence of dental caries compared with those who had been colonised later in childhood (Köhler et al., 1988). Prolonged infection with high levels of mutans streptococci had also been associated with increased levels of dental caries in both the primary and permanent teeth (Straetemans et al., 1998).

By obtaining plaque samples from twins and their parents and siblings, it was aimed to find out whether mutans streptococci were acquired from both mothers and fathers, or predominantly from mothers as reported in most previous studies. Another aim was to determine whether acquisition of mutans streptococci was associated with emergence of particular primary teeth, and whether there was any relationship with subsequent caries experience. A further question that we wanted to answer, using DNA fingerprinting techniques, was whether monozygotic and dizygotic pairs of twins harboured the same or different strains of mutans streptococci.

The plan was for the parents of the twins to record the timing of emergence of all the primary teeth in their twins. A pilot study was carried out to ensure that the recording sheets we were planning to use, and also the surveys about the health and habits of the twins and their parents, were clear and unambiguous. The pilot study also enabled us to confirm that the families could follow our instructions for recording the emergence of teeth, as well as being able to collect samples of cheek cells for zygosity testing and plaque samples for microbiological assessment. It was planned to collect plaque samples every three months from the twins and every twelve months from parents and other siblings. We also checked that the transportation of these records to our laboratory was efficient and effective.

The recruiting phase of the study involved contacting mothers-to-be or mothers of newborn twins throughout Australia and obtaining their permission to participate in the study. Families were recruited through the NHMRC Twin Registry in Melbourne and we also scanned through the birth columns of Australian newspapers to identify newly born twins. The parents of the twins who agreed to participate were asked to complete an initial questionnaire that provided information on the pregnancy, maternal habits (such as smoking and drinking alcohol), birthweight

Cohort 3 – Tooth emergence and oral health in Australian twins

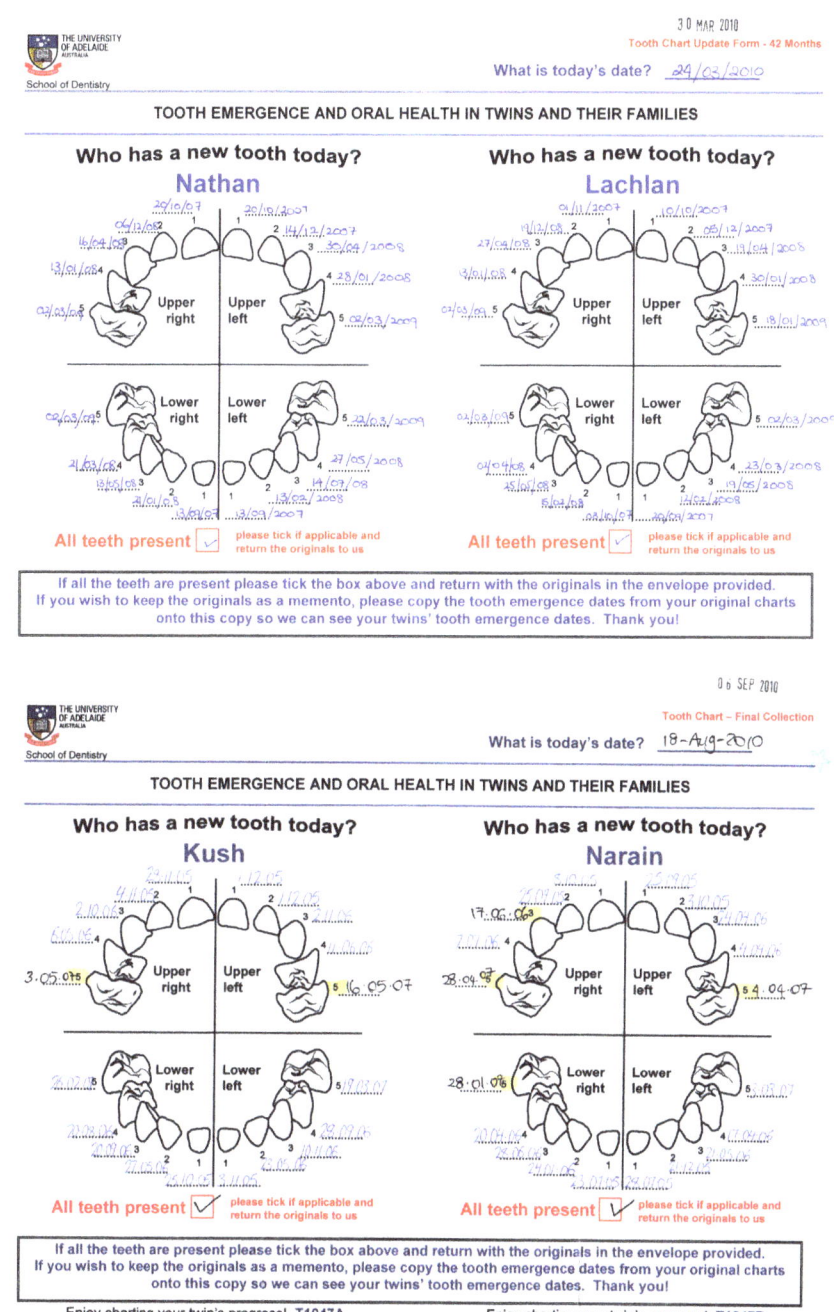

Figure 6.3
Recording sheets for tooth emergence, including a pair of monozygotic twins (above) and a pair of same-sex dizygotic twins (below).

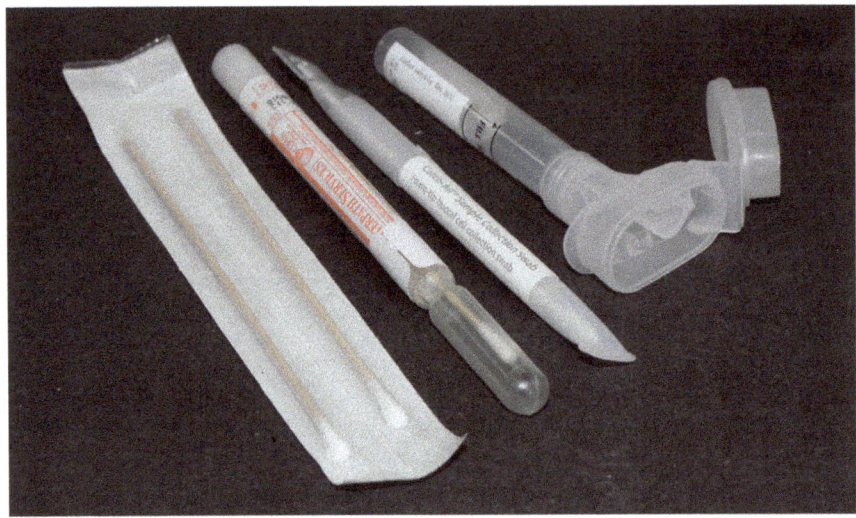

Figure 6.4
Examples of the collection kits for dental plaque, buccal cells and saliva sent to families.

and length of the twins, and any illnesses. Parents were also given instructions and forms (by email and hard copy) to record the times at which each of the twenty primary teeth appeared in their twins' mouths. We asked the parents to obtain cheek cells of their twins for subsequent DNA analysis and zygosity testing, too, as well as plaque samples for assessment of oral mutans streptococci levels and presence of other microbes.

Scanning the birth columns of the Australian newspapers to look for births of twins has proved to be a very fruitful method for recruiting families of twins to Cohort 3, and our honorary research assistant, Ruth Rogers, has worked tirelessly to identify potential participants.

It was decided to give the parents another questionnaire when the twins were around 12 months old. This survey focused on postnatal issues, including information about any illnesses, medications, dietary habits, teething problems, and thumb- and finger-sucking habits. Measurements of the twins' weight and height were also obtained. The parents' recordings of tooth emergence were checked by clinically examining sub-samples of the twins. These examinations confirmed the validity of the records being obtained (Hughes et al., 2007).

Cohort 3 – Tooth emergence and oral health in Australian twins

The vagaries of the grant funding process

In 2007, we submitted an application to the NHMRC for a continuation of funding for 2008-10, but our application was not successful. This represented a major blow to our research momentum, as we were in the middle of a longitudinal study. During the first two years of the project we had recruited over 400 pairs of twins and their families Australia-wide, and had also commenced some analyses and submitted papers for publication. The negative outcome of our application was a major shock, given that no other study of this type had been undertaken previously, and given that the reviewers' comments were all very positive. The inclusion of twins and the use of a longitudinal study design were enabling us to examine how an individual's genotype, as well as his/her environment, acted upon both the timing and sequence of tooth emergence and the likelihood of suffering dental decay from an early age. Although a group of researchers in the USA was investigating the role of genetic factors in the development of dental caries in Brazilian twins (Bretz et al., 2005a,b), they were focusing neither on tooth emergence nor on how the timing of tooth emergence was associated with colonisation with mutans streptococci.

With limited funding, progress on our study slowed considerably, although we managed to keep the record collection ticking over. A grant of $AUS50 000 from the Financial Markets Foundation for Children proved to be a lifeline for our study, enabling us to continue to collect records from twins and their families; and our total sample increased to over 600 families Australia-wide. We were also able to compile and begin to administer a third questionnaire to gather more information on oral hygiene, diet and dental disease in our cohort.

Getting beaten to the punch

We were well aware at the time of the major advances occurring in the field of molecular genetics and the potential of genome-wide scanning approaches to identify genes contributing to variation in complex multifactorial disorders and diseases, such as hypertension and diabetes. We submitted grant applications to the NHMRC to use linkage and association approaches to identify genes for dental development, but our applications were unsuccessful.

Table 6.1
Topics included in the questionnaires filled out by families of twins.

Questionnaire Headings	Questions relating to
Feeding Practice	Breast- or bottle-fed, feeding times
Teeth and Oral Health Care	Tooth loss
	Tooth-brushing habits
	Dentist visits and teeth condition
	Teething
	Thumb-sucking habits
	Persons with whom twins spend most time
Diet	Food most commonly eaten
General Health and Medical History	Twins' height, weight and past illnesses
Smoking and Drinking	Parents' smoking and drinking habits
Parents' Oral Health and Health Care	Tooth-brushing habits
	Medication taken
	Dental visits and condition of teeth
Optional	Tooth charts to record the condition of twins' and parents' teeth

In 2010, the findings of a genome-wide association study (GWAS) of the timing of primary tooth emergence in two large cohorts of children were published (Pillas et al., 2010). The authors referred to our work, which had shown a very strong genetic influence on the timing of emergence of the primary teeth (high heritability), but we were very disappointed that we had not been the first group to report on which genes seemed to affect tooth emergence.

Interestingly, five genetic loci were identified in the above-mentioned GWAS as being involved in human dental development, with four of these also being implicated in the development of cancer, while another was associated with occlusal anomalies in the permanent dentition that required orthodontic treatment in later life. This latter finding provided strong support for our contention that improved understanding of the genetic, environmental and epigenetic influences on human primary tooth emergence is needed to inform the clinical management of orthodontic problems affecting not only the primary teeth but also the permanent teeth.

In addition to the GWAS of primary tooth emergence mentioned earlier, a GWAS of permanent tooth emergence was carried out subsequently by an international team of researchers (Pillas et al., 2010; Geller et al., 2011). In the study of primary tooth emergence, a variant of the *HOXB* gene cluster was associated with alterations in dental occlusion of those study subjects who required orthodontic treatment in later life (Pillas et al., 2010). The *HOX* genes are a group of regulator genes that have been conserved throughout the course of vertebrate evolution. They are involved in controlling the arrangement of body parts during development, including patterning effects within the dentition — for example, the formation of incisors, canines and molars in their correct positions within the dental arches.

Meanwhile, in the study of permanent tooth emergence, two identified loci associated with stature and breast cancer were consistent with those identified for primary tooth emergence, but the other loci had not been identified previously (Geller et al., 2011).

In a recent study, a group of international researchers carried out a genome-wide association study of facial morphology in nearly 10 000 individuals of European descent, using 3D magnetic resonance images and 2D portrait images. Five independent genetic loci were identified which were associated with different facial phenotypes, suggesting that five candidate genes are involved in the determination of facial morphology. Three of the candidate genes, namely *PAX3*, *PRDM16* and *TP63*, have been implicated previously in craniofacial development, whereas the other two had not been identified as being directly involved in craniofacial development in the past (Liu et al., 2012).

Genome-wide association studies in dentistry are now helping to identify which particular genes are associated with dental development and oral health (Stanley et al., 2014). Although these large-scale, multi-centre projects are still in their infancy in dentistry, dental researchers have the advantage of being able to draw on the experiences of geneticists and medical researchers, who have now overcome many of the inherent difficulties and limitations of genome-wide association studies. Traditionally, genome-wide association studies have been based on unrelated case/control populations, but underlying stratification in the populations may lead to spurious or misleading associations. By including family groupings in these types of studies, particularly twins, some of the problems of population stratification can be overcome (Hughes and Townsend, 2013).

Twin Studies

AN EXCITING NEW COLLABORATION

Although the outcome of our NHMRC grant application in 2007 was a major disappointment, the year marked the beginning of an exciting new and continuing collaboration involving our studies of twins. Grant Townsend spent a period of sabbatical leave in Liverpool with Professor Alan Brook and his research team, who had recently relocated from Sheffield. Over 200 sets of vacuum-formed plastic impressions had been made of selected dental models of twins in Adelaide and these were then shipped to Liverpool, where they were poured up in stone. This provided a duplicate set of dental models that could then be studied in Liverpool. Alan Brook and Richard Smith had set up state-of-the-art imaging equipment, both 2D and 3D, to enable novel measurements of the teeth to be made, including areas, perimeters and volumes.

During this time, a workshop was held in Liverpool to establish an International Collaborating Centre in Oro-facial Genetics and Development, with Alan Brook, Lassi Alvesalo and Grant Townsend as co-directors. A special issue of the journal *Archives of Oral Biology* was subsequently published, containing refereed papers arising from the workshop (Brook, 2009). The aim of the International Collaborating Centre was to bring together colleagues from different centres around the world who were using different approaches, so that existing collaborations could be developed further and new collaborations established.

It was decided to purchase similar imaging equipment to that in Liverpool for our laboratory in Adelaide so that we could ensure a standardised approach to future studies. Alan Brook then came to Adelaide to consolidate the links that had been established. Indeed, he is now spending most of his time in Adelaide as an Adjunct Professor in the School of Dentistry, and as a key member of our research group. The Collaborating Centre has been developed as a Collaborating Network, and a special issue of the *Australian Dental Journal,* edited by Grant Townsend and Alan Brook, which contains several papers from members of the Craniofacial Biology Research Group and the International Collaborating Network, was published in June 2014 (Townsend and Brook, 2014).

Cohort 3 – Tooth emergence and oral health in Australian twins

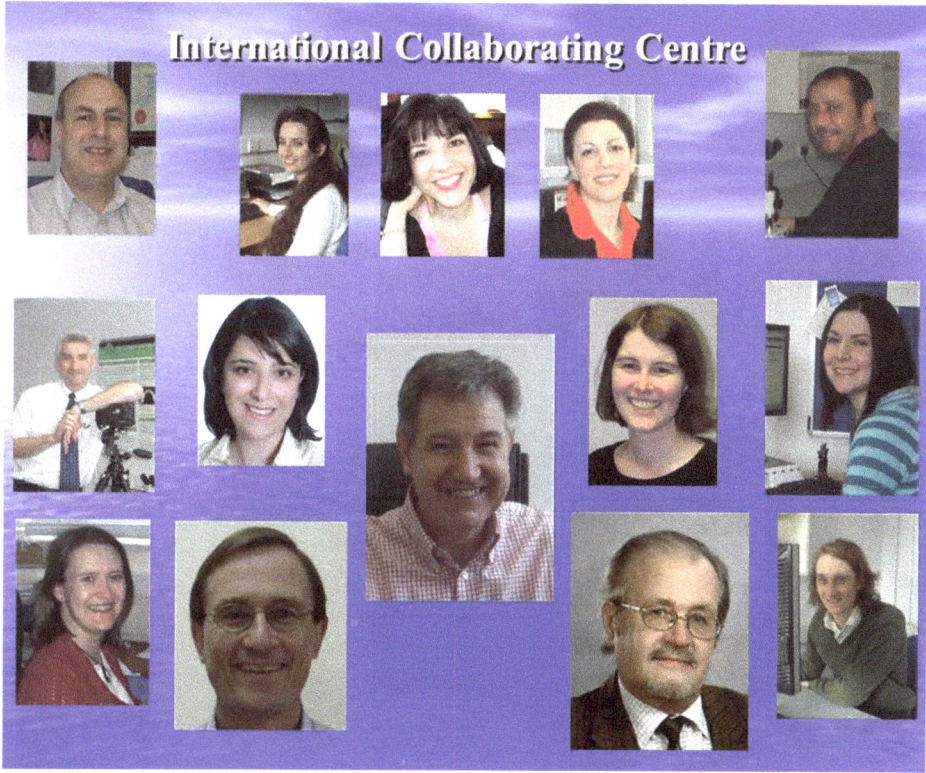

Figure 6.5
Some of the initial members of the International Collaborating Centre in Oro-facial Genetics and Development, with Professor Alan Brook in the centre.

Developments in epigenetics

The field of epigenetics has developed exponentially over the past decade or so, but epigenetics is not a new concept. Phenotypic discordance in monozygotic co-twins — that is, differences in appearance of various features between pairs of monozygotic twins — was traditionally interpreted as indicating the influence of environmental factors on the feature or trait being investigated. However, more recently, evidence has accumulated that epigenetic modifications of DNA, such as methylation of DNA, can influence the expression of genes.

Although molecular geneticists have tended to focus on processes such as the methylation and acetylation of segments of DNA when referring to the term 'epigenetics', we have used a broader interpretation of the term, following on from the pioneering work of Conrad Waddington (1957). We consider that the term 'epigenetics' can be used to refer to all of the processes by which the genotype gives rise to the phenotype (Townsend et al., 2009). For example, epigenetic effects may involve modification of DNA through methylation or alteration in histone packaging through acetylation, but they may also refer to the interactive processes that occur between cells at the local tissue level during development (Williams et al., 2014).

Waddington provided a fascinating visual metaphor to illustrate the concept of an 'epigenetic landscape', representing the processes by which cells make decisions during development. He likened the different stages of cellular decision-making during development to a ball rolling down an undulating landscape of interconnecting hills and valleys. At various stages on this landscape, the ball (or cell) could take specific permitted trajectories that would lead to different outcomes or cellular fates. We have extended this metaphor to include the influence of epigenetic processes on a pair of monozygotic twins (Figure 6.6).

This metaphor would seem to be very appropriate when considering the developmental processes involved in odontogenesis, or tooth formation. Minor variations in the timing and/or spatial relationships of interacting cells have the potential to lead to quite different phenotypic outcomes — for example, the absence of a tooth rather than its presence, or the development of an extra tooth. Small differences in the epigenetic landscape between right and left sides of the dentition may also lead to distinct or subtle differences in the morphology of antimeric teeth (that is, corresponding teeth on opposite sides of the dental arch). We would contend that differences in the epigenetic landscape between monozygotic co-twins are likely to account for some of the differences in dental phenotypes we have observed in these twin pairs.

Waddington's concept of epigenetics is compatible with the apparent dynamic self-organising nature of tooth formation (also referred to as odontogenesis), which leads to the 'unfolding' of each tooth's morphology. More recently, with our colleague Professor Alan Brook, we have been investigating the development of teeth as an example of a Complex Adaptive System (Brook et al., 2014).

Studies of epigenetic differences between monozygotic twin pairs are now helping to explain phenotypic differences between monozygotic co-twins. Mario Fraga and colleagues (2005) assessed the extent of two important epigenetic

Cohort 3 – Tooth emergence and oral health in Australian twins

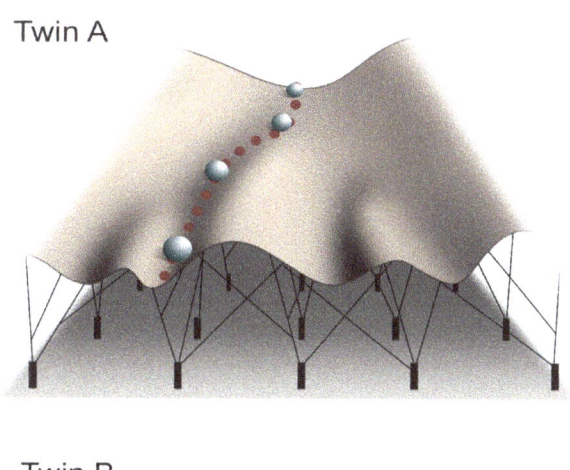

Twin A

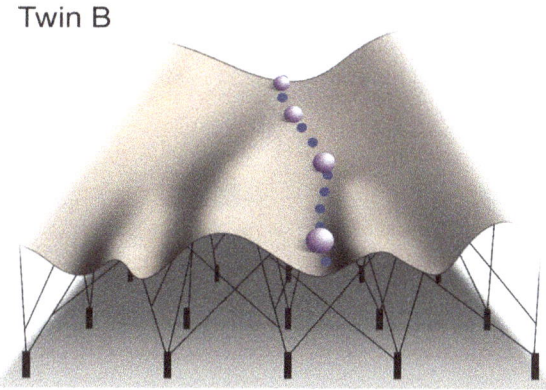

Twin B

Figure 6.6
Waddington's epigenetic landscape is a metaphor for how gene regulation modulates development. Imagine a number of marbles rolling down a hill towards a wall. The marbles will compete for the grooves on the slope, and the ridges between the grooves represent the increasing irreversibility of cell type differentiation. Each marble will come to rest at the lowest possible point, representing eventual cell fates, or tissue types. Reproduced with permission from the *Australian Dental Journal* (Hughes et al., 2014).

modifications, DNA methylation and histone acetylation, in the genomes of forty pairs of monozygotic twins. They found that the epigenetic profiles of monozygotic co-twins were almost identical in 65 per cent of the twin pairs, whereas there were significant differences in the other 35 per cent of twin pairs. Intriguingly, the amount of epigenetic difference was directly related to the age of the twins, as well as to the amount of time co-twins had spent apart. The epigenetic differences between co-twins were also greater in those pairs who had different medical histories. These findings may explain why some MZ co-twins seem to become less alike with age. They also suggest that environmental disturbances are likely to contribute to epigenetic changes that accumulate over time. A recent review by Jordana Bell and Tim Spector (2011) provides further details about how large-scale epigenetic studies of twins promise to provide important insights into the way that genetic, environmental and stochastic (random) factors influence epigenetics and, in turn, variation of complex traits.

Research following the completion of the Human Genome Project has demonstrated that the aetiology of complex diseases cannot be explained by genetics alone. Much research is now looking at epigenetics in an effort to elucidate how the environment interacts with our genes to bring a phenotype or disease process into being. One aspect of current research in the Craniofacial Biology Research Group involves investigating whether a discordant epigenetic profile may be associated with discordant expression of dental developmental anomalies in Australian monozygotic twins. We have subjected sixty DNA samples from thirty monozygotic twin pairs to epigenetic analysis (genome-wide microarray methylation profiling). A control group of concordant monozygotic pairs was compared with a group of discordant pairs for missing and extra teeth. All groups were ascertained across a broad range of tooth sizes, and an approximately equal distribution of males and females was selected.

DNA samples were taken at the time of phenotyping, approximately twenty years ago. Although a degree of degradation was evident, our samples are still of high quality. Preliminary results have shown that there is a substantial degree of discordance in epigenetic profiles between many monozygotic twin pairs, and that this discordance may be greater for twins with discordant dentitions. Our preliminary analysis suggests that, at a genome-wide level, there may be an influence of methylation status on tooth formation, manifesting in variation in the presence or absence of teeth. Further analyses are required to investigate effects on tooth size, and more sophisticated site-specific analyses are also required to investigate specific genes. Epigenetics research is now being applied in several areas of dentistry, and promises to have far-reaching clinical implications in the future (Williams et al., 2014).

Cohort 3 – Tooth emergence and oral health in Australian twins

Next-generation sequencing

The advent of next-generation sequencing methods is providing enormous power to genetically characterise diverse biological samples without needing any prior information about the actual DNA sequences present. In collaboration with Dr Christina Adler and Professor Neil Hunter at the University of Sydney, we are now sequencing microbial DNA extracted from the dental plaque samples being collected from the twins and family members in Cohort 3. The depth of sequencing provided by next-generation methods enables sensitive detection and discrimination of a wide diversity of microbes. In addition, this method also enables the relative abundance of different bacterial components of the sequenced microbial community to be determined.

Our aim, using these state-of-the-art methods, is to demonstrate the degree to which genetic and environmental factors influence variation in the oral microbiota. We have, therefore, extended our microbiological studies to include other bacteria apart from mutans streptococci.

The current consensus is that dental decay is caused by a microbial shift in oral biofilms (dental plaque) due to carbohydrate consumption, leading to demineralisation of the tooth surface. This hypothesis is referred to as the 'extended ecological plaque hypothesis' (Takahashi and Nyvad, 2008). It views dental plaque as being composed of a dynamic microbial ecosystem in which there are many different bacteria, with the non-mutans bacteria being key organisms in maintaining dynamic stability. With increasing numbers of non-mutans bacteria that can thrive in a low-pH environment, the microbial composition of the plaque can become destabilised, leading to an increase in mutans streptococci that have the potential to promote the development of carious lesions.

This hypothesis, however, does not consider the role of host genetic factors in the development of dental caries — an effect we demonstrated through our study of oral microbiota in twins belonging to Cohort 3 (approximately 300 monozygotic and 300 dizygotic twin pairs). Furthermore, it is unclear whether caries is associated with an enrichment of a small number of cariogenic (decay-producing) species or a change in the overall structure of the oral microbiota. As a result, it is unclear exactly how the oral bacteria of a child with dental decay differ from those of a healthy individual.

Figure 6.7 shows an intra-oral photograph of one member of a pair of monozygotic twins enrolled in Cohort 3 who shows extensive dental decay. One focus of our current research is to record the expression of dental decay in pairs of monozygotic twins, as we have already noted examples where the patterns of expression are very similar (concordant) and other examples where they differ considerably (that is, they are discordant). We have also noted discordance in expression of other dental features in monozygotic twin pairs — for example, in tooth emergence and also gingival health.

Figure 6.8 shows the anterior teeth of a pair of monozygotic twins enrolled in Cohort 3. Twin A displays accumulation of dental plaque around the necks of the

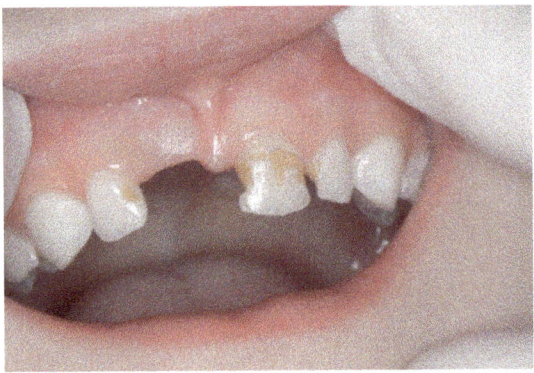

Figure 6.7
An example of extensive dental decay affecting the anterior primary teeth of one of the twins enrolled in Cohort 3.

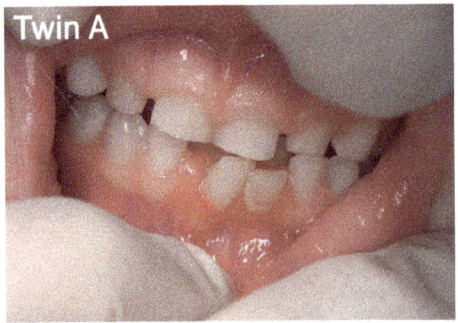 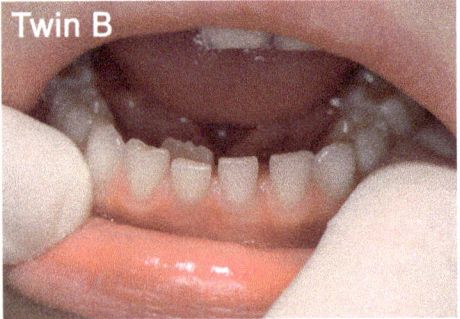

Figure 6.8
Different expressions of dental problems in a pair of monozygotic twins.

primary lower left incisors associated with gingival inflammation. These teeth are loose, whereas Twin B has a permanent lower central incisor erupting behind the retained primary incisor.

A new NHMRC grant

An application to the NHMRC by Christina Adler, Toby Hughes, Grant Townsend and Manish Arora for a research project entitled 'Determining how genetic and environmental factors influence the developing oral microbiota and drive disease in early childhood' was successful in receiving funding and commenced in 2014. Christina Adler undertook her PhD with Professor Alan Cooper and his group in the Centre for Ancient DNA at the University of Adelaide, and we have established a collaboration with them to explore the oral microbiome of prehistoric humans, based on DNA analysis of dental calculus, also referred to as tartar. After her PhD, Christina took up an academic position in the Dental School at the University of Sydney.

A key focus of this new project is to extend our understanding of childhood caries by revealing how genetic, epigenetic and environmental factors drive variation in the composition of the developing oral microbiota through in-depth genetic analyses. Using approaches described in a recent paper in *Nature Genetics* (Adler et al., 2013), it is planned to provide a more sophisticated understanding of how the whole oral microbial community contributes to the maintenance of oral health and also to the development of dental decay.

Two of the research questions we are addressing are:

1. Is dental caries associated with the enrichment of a few cariogenic species or a range of species that cause a change in the overall community structure of the oral microbiota?

2. Are the oral microbial species that are enriched in caries as well as in health influenced mainly by environmental or genetic factors?

The human mouth contains between 10^2 and 10^3 different species of bacteria that can contribute to both health and disease. It is known that colonisation of the mouth with these different types of bacteria commences at birth, and that the composition of the oral microflora (or oral microbiota) is influenced by environmental influences during infancy, such as diet and the use of antibiotics. Generally, the microbiota tend to reach stable levels by early childhood.

Apart from environmental influences, it is suspected that each individual's genetic make-up (their genotype) plays a role in determining the overall composition of the oral microbiota, as family members have been shown to have more similar microbial profiles than non-related individuals. Heritable components of the oral microbiota are thought to play a role in the development of dental decay, with studies showing that the similarity of caries experience in monozygotic co-twins is greater than that in dizygotic co-twins. In fact, estimates of heritability for dental caries experience range from 30 per cent to 60 per cent (Boraas et al., 1988; Wang et al., 2010). However, it is still unclear what the relative contributions of genetic and environmental influences are to observed variation in the composition of the oral microbiota, and this is one of the key questions we are addressing from both anthropological and genetic viewpoints (Kaidonis and Townsend, 2015).

Collection of plaque and saliva samples from Cohort 3 is ongoing, as well as clinical examinations to detect evidence of dental caries and developmental abnormalities of the teeth and oral soft tissues (Figure 6.9).

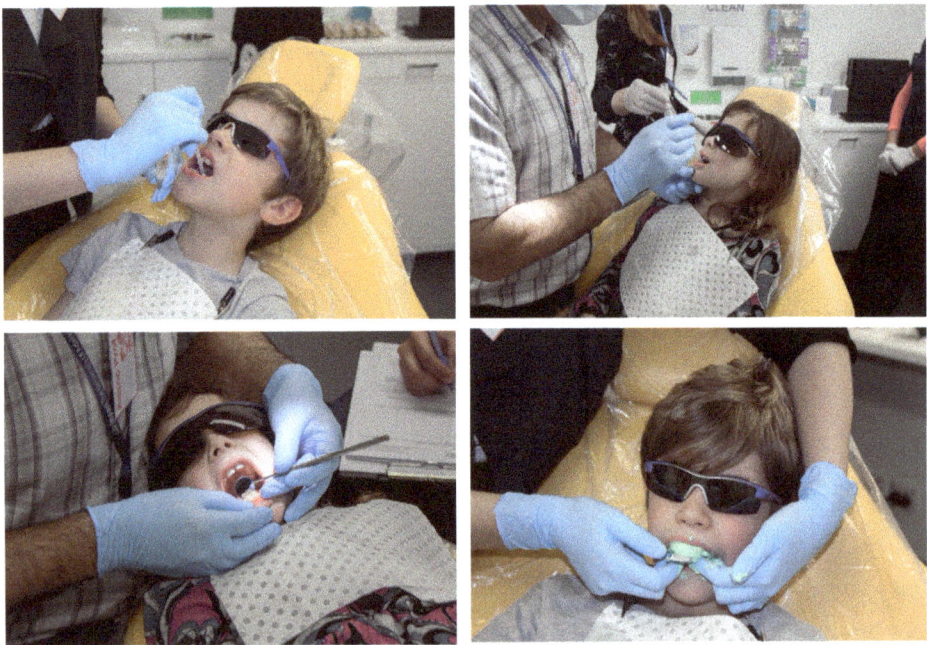

Figure 6.9
Clinical examinations of twins.

Cohort 3 – Tooth emergence and oral health in Australian twins

Apart from the new records being collected from the participants in Cohort 3, including plaque and saliva samples and buccal cells for epigenetic testing, we are continuing to obtain dental impressions to enable stone models of the teeth to be constructed. We are also obtaining fingerprints, carrying out laterality tests and recording heights and weights. Some other new recordings being obtained in collaboration with colleagues in Melbourne include blood pressure readings. Figure 6.10 shows various records being obtained from twins in Cohort 3.

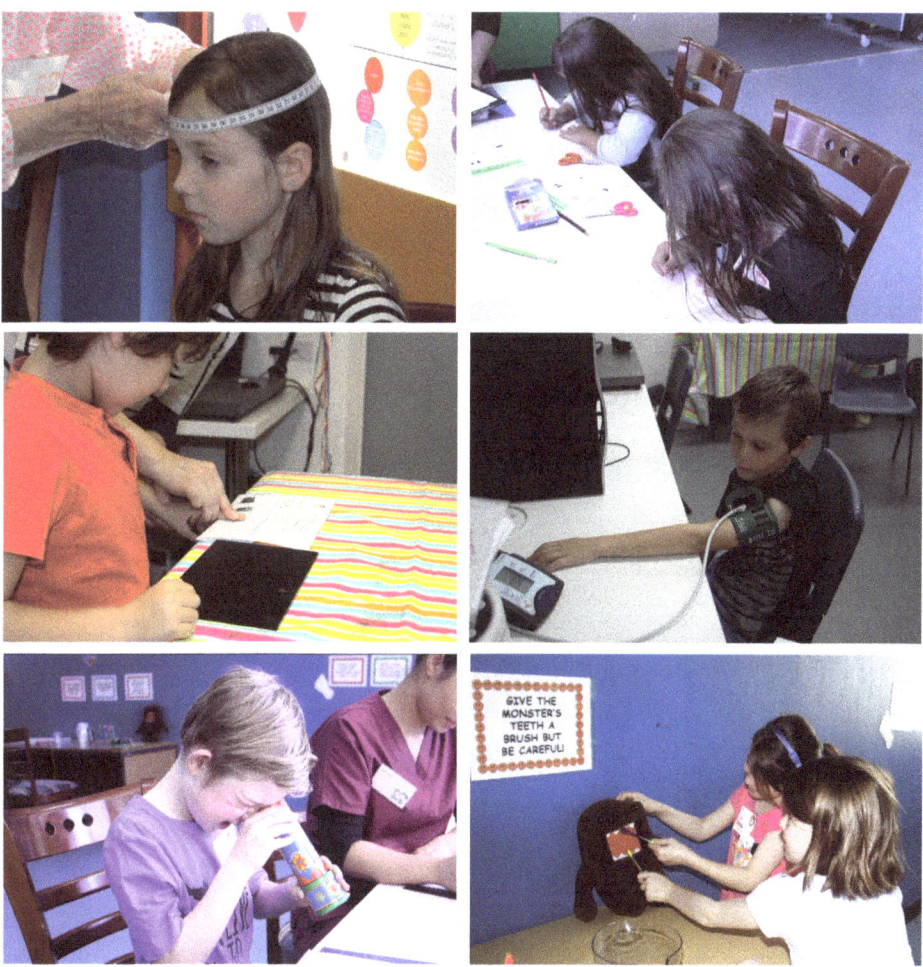

Figure 6.10
Various tests and measurements are performed during the visits.

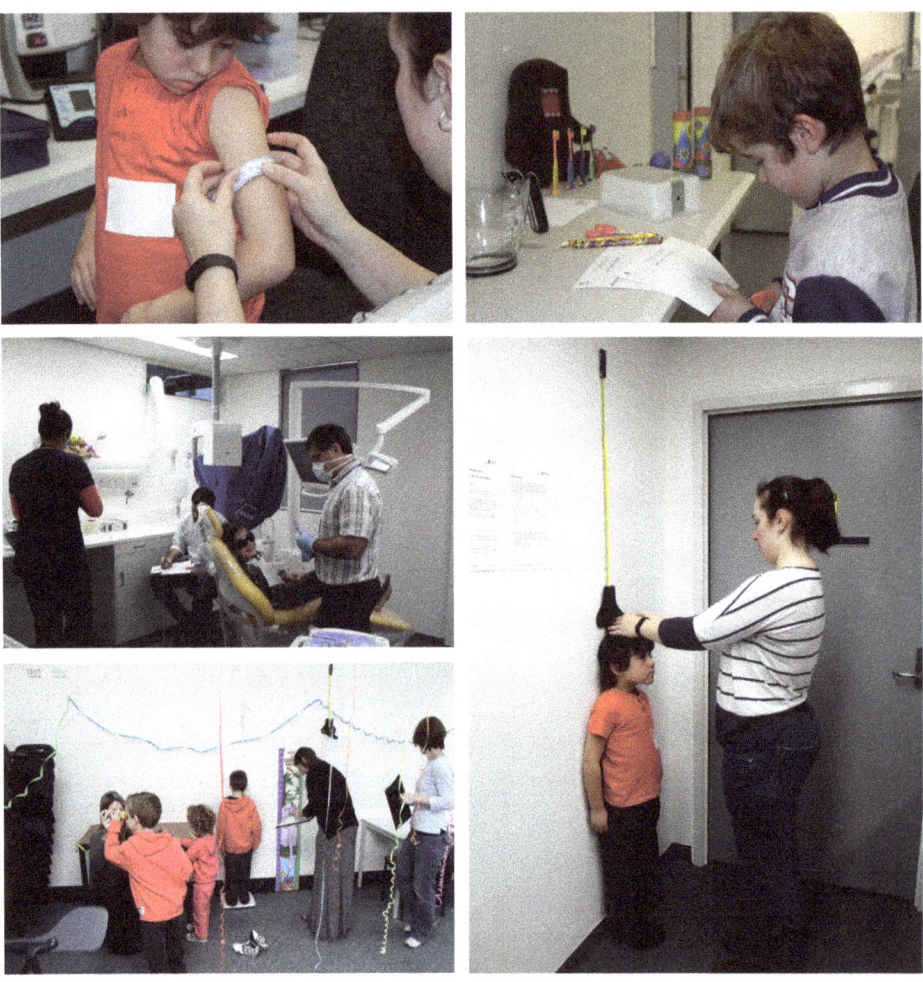

Figure 6.10 continued.

We have now reached a stage where children of twins who were enrolled in our second cohort are involved in Cohort 3 (Figure 6.11).

THE FUTURE

With the development of new equipment for measuring teeth and components of teeth, it is now becoming possible to define more biologically meaningful dental phenotypes. Following on from the establishment of the International Collaborating Network in Oro-facial Genetics and Development in Liverpool in 2007, we have now

Cohort 3 – Tooth emergence and oral health in Australian twins

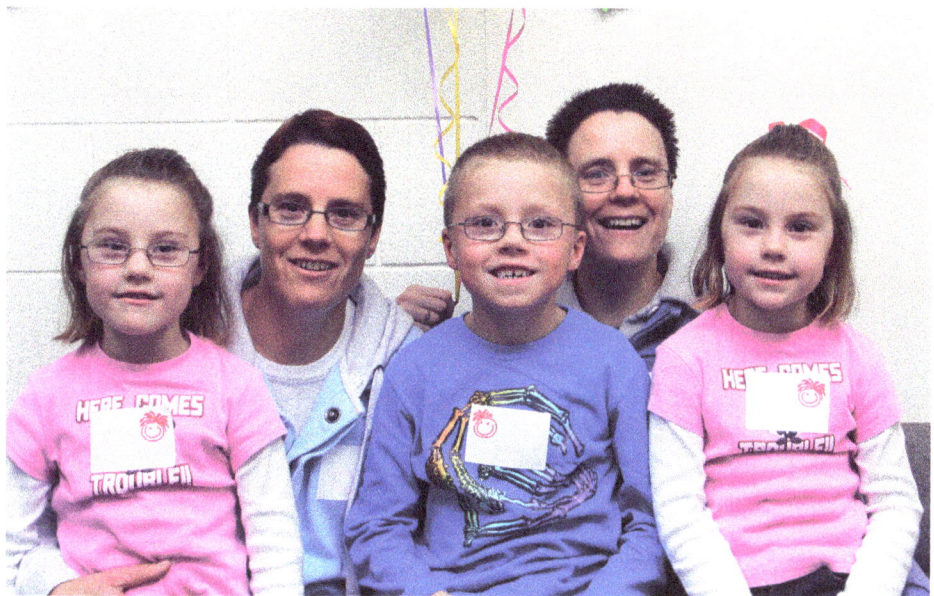

Figure 6.11
Two generations of twins enrolled in our ongoing studies. The twins who are seated behind participated in Cohort 2, and the children in front are the twin monozygotic daughters and son of one of the twins, who are now participating in Cohort 3.

set up two-dimensional (2D) and three-dimensional (3D) imaging equipment in our laboratory in Adelaide. We have confirmed that these systems have high accuracy and reliability, and research projects to clarify how genetic, epigenetic and environmental factors contribute to morphological variation within the dentition are both underway and planned. Figure 6.12 shows how 2D imaging enables defects in enamel to be quantified from study models.

Figure 6.13 shows 3D models of teeth and dental arches generated by a laser scanner.

Advances in the fields of micro- and nano-imaging are also opening up new avenues to explore the internal structure of teeth, as well as their physical and chemical properties. We have now collected a large number of exfoliated (shed) primary teeth, which are providing an opportunity to further study tooth structure (Figure 6.14).

Figure 6.15 shows 3D micro-CT images of teeth from a pair of monozygotic twins where there is evidence of Carabelli trait at the dentino-enamel junction as well

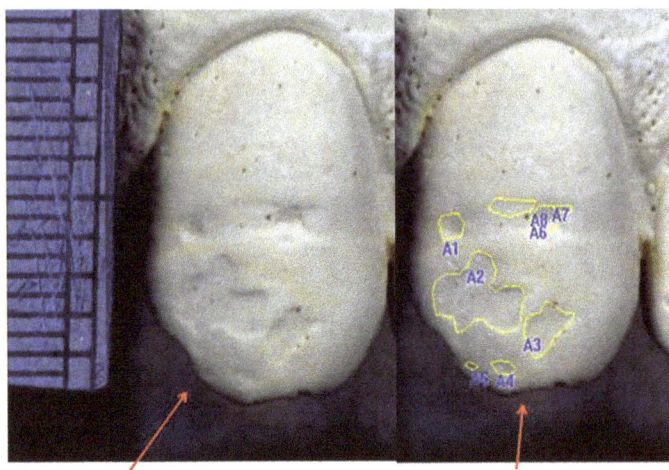

Digital 2D image of an upper incisor demonstrating enamel hypoplasia

Subsequent defects isolated for area measurement

Figure 6.12
2D imaging of enamel defects. Reproduced with permission from the *Australian Dental Journal* (Yong et al., 2014).

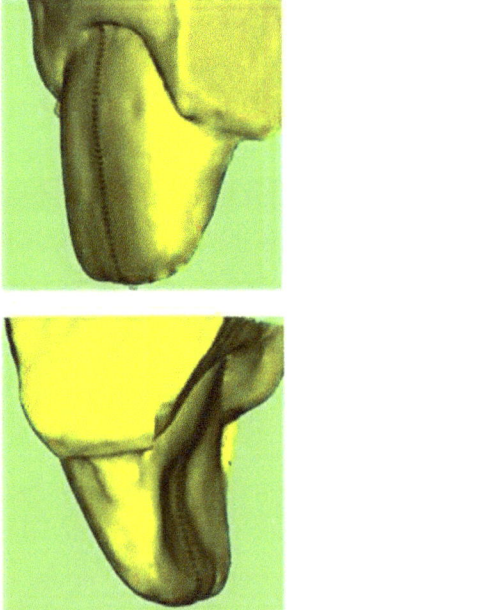
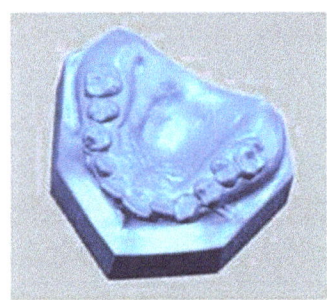
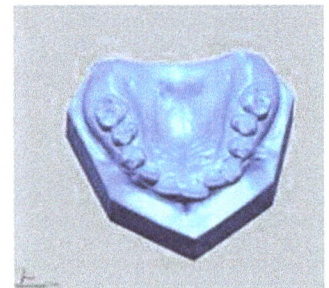

Figure 6.13
3D models of teeth (Townsend et al., 2012).

Cohort 3 – Tooth emergence and oral health in Australian twins

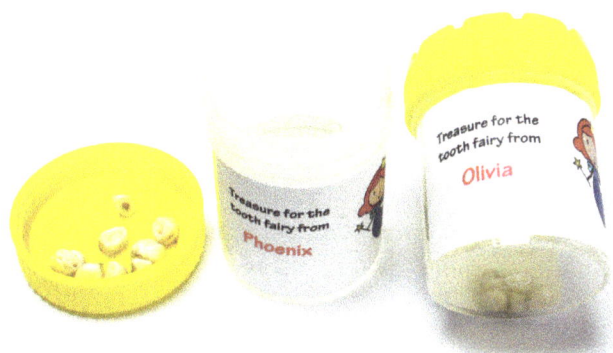

Figure 6.14
Exfoliated primary teeth from a pair of twins.

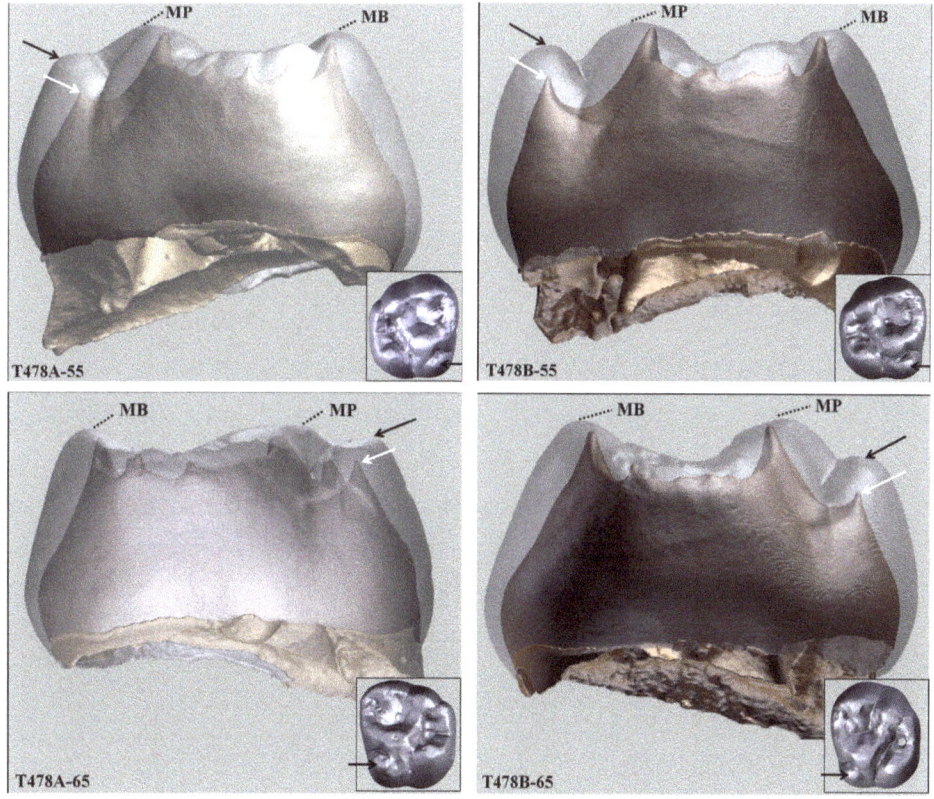

Figure 6.15
3D micro-CT images of teeth from a pair of monozygotic twins. The 3D models were generated by Dr Jeremy Deverell at the South Australian node of the Australian National Fabrication Facility under the National Collaborative Research Infrastructure Strategy. Reproduced with permission from the *Australian Dental Journal* (Hughes et al., 2014).

as on the enamel surface. Planned studies based on these types of images offer great promise to link observed expression of dental features on the external surfaces of teeth to events occurring at the site of the future dentino-enamel junction, where the developing tooth folds to produce its crown shape.

We continue to pursue new opportunities to undertake collaborative, multi-centre research in orofacial growth and development and oral health. Some recent examples include:

- a grant application to the NIH with Professor Walter Bretz from New York University to analyse genes associated with salivary proteins in two national twin cohorts, one from Brazil and one from our Cohort 3 from Australia
- early dialogue to undertake GWAS for orofacial phenotypes in a consortium of twin cohorts, including Cohorts 1, 2 and 3 from our group, various twin cohorts from Professor Nick Martin's genetic epidemiology group at the Queensland Institute of Medical Research, and several twin cohorts from Professor Alex Vieira's group at the University of Pittsburgh
- a collaborative effort between our group, Associate Professor Jeff Craig's group at the Melbourne Children's Research Institute and the J Craig Venter Institute in the USA to undertake next-generation sequencing of DNA and RNA from oral microbiome samples of twins
- two new initiatives with dental anthropologists from the USA, Kathleen Paul and Richard Scott. Paul will spend time in Adelaide examining dental models of twins to test the performance of several dental features in reconstructing genetic relationships for bioarcheological applications. Scott will work on a new edition of the classic text '*The Anthropology of Modern Human Teeth*' in Adelaide with Grant Townsend, and will examine the twins' dental models.

SOME OF THE KEY FINDINGS RELATING TO COHORT 3

1. Accurate and up-to-date data on the timing and sequence of tooth emergence are important for researchers, clinicians and parents. Based on data collected from Cohort 3, updated tables have been produced for the timing and sequence of primary tooth emergence in Australian children.

The first and last primary teeth emerged, on average, at 8.6 months and 27.9 months, respectively. The order of emergence, based on average values, was central incisor, lateral incisor, first molar canine, and second molar. However, there was considerable variation in the sequence of emergence between individuals. Around 35 per cent of all corresponding teeth on opposite sides of the arch emerged within two weeks of each other. These findings indicate that primary tooth emergence is occurring later than reported previously for Australian children but the sequence has remained the same. Another study of the patterns of asymmetry in primary tooth emergence showed relatively low levels of fluctuating asymmetry throughout the dentition (minor differences between right and left sides without any tendency for one side to be consistently earlier in emergence than the other), with the maxillary and mandibular lateral incisors displaying the highest values (Mihailidis et al., 2009; Woodroffe et al., 2010).

2. Our finding that there is a very high genetic influence on variation in primary tooth emergence in Australian twins was the first report to be published based on sophisticated genetic modelling methods and it spurred on the race to identify the genes associated with tooth eruption using genome-wide association studies (Hughes et al., 2007; Bockmann et al., 2010).

3. A paper entitled 'Genetic and environmental influences on human dental variation: a critical evaluation of studies involving twins', arising from the International Workshop on Oral Growth and Development, which was held in November 2007 in Liverpool, was published in a special issue of *Archives of Oral Biology* in 2009. This paper discusses the different methods of analysis which can be carried out using data derived from twins, and considers the advantages and disadvantages of these different approaches. Results from our studies of Cohorts 1, 2 and 3 are summarised and some of the opportunities for future research explored (Townsend et al., 2009).

4. In a study of primary tooth emergence and timing of oral colonisation of *Streptococcus mutans*, it was found that approximately 20 per cent of monozygotic twin pairs were discordant (that is, they differed) for the timing of colonisation, in terms of whether colonisation occurred

before or after the first primary tooth had emerged. This suggests that environmental or epigenetic factors are likely to influence the timing of tooth emergence, or the colonisation by *Streptococcus mutans*, or both of these variables. These findings provide hope that it may be possible to develop strategies to prevent or delay infection of children with *Streptococcus mutans* and, therefore, to reduce the likelihood of future dental disease — in other words, dental decay (Bockmann et al., 2011).

5. Two areas of research that we have pursued in recent times have been those of phenomics and epigenetics. We believe that these areas will become increasingly important in the future. Recently, Grant Townsend and Alan Brook edited a special issue of the *Australian Dental Journal* entitled: 'The face, the future, and dental practice: how research in craniofacial biology will influence patient care'. This issue includes several papers that refer to our ongoing studies of Australian twins, including papers that are devoted to the topics of dental phenomics and epigenetics. Readers are directed to this volume if they would like to learn more about these topics (Townsend and Brook, 2014; Hughes et al., 2014; Williams et al., 2014; Yong et al., 2014).

References

Adler CJ, Dobney K, Weyrich LS, Kaidonis J, Walker AW, Haak W, et al. (2013). Sequencing ancient calcified dental plaque shows changes in oral microbiota with dietary shifts of the Neolithic and Industrial revolutions. *Nat Genet* 45:450-455.

Armfield JM, Spencer AJ, Brennan DS (2009). Dental health of Australia's teenagers and pre-teen children: the Child Dental Health Survey, Australia 2003-04. *Dental statistics and research series no. 52. Cat. no. DEN 199.* Canberra: Australian Institute of Health and Welfare.

Bell JT, Spector TD (2011). A twin approach to unravelling epigenetics. *Trends Genet* 27:116-125.

Bockmann MR, Harris AV, Bennett CN, Odeh R, Hughes TE, Townsend GC (2011). Timing of colonization of caries-producing bacteria: an approach based on studying monozygotic twin pairs. *Int J Dent* Article ID 571573, 7 pages, doi:10.1155/2011/571573. Accessed 19 May 2015.

Bockmann MR, Hughes TE, Townsend GC (2010). Genetic modeling of primary tooth emergence: a study of Australian twins. *Twin Res Hum Genet* 13:573-581.

Boraas JC, Messer LB, Till MJ (1988). A genetic contribution to dental caries, occlusion, and morphology as demonstrated by twins reared apart. *J Dent Res* 67:1150-1155.

Bretz WA, Corby PM, Hart TC, Costa S, Coelho MQ, Weyant RJ, et al. (2005a). Dental caries and microbial acid production in twins. *Caries Res* 39:168-172.

Bretz WA, Corby PM, Schork NJ, Robinson MT, Coelho M, Costa S, et al. (2005b). Longitudinal analysis of heritability for dental caries traits. *J Dent Res* 84:1047-1051.

Brook AH (2009). Editorial. Research collaborative initiative. *Arch Oral Biol* 54S:S1-S2.

Brook AH, Brook O'Donnell M, Hone A, Hart E, Hughes TE, Smith R, et al. (2014). General and craniofacial development are complex adaptive processes influenced by diversity. *Aust Dent J* 59 (1 Suppl):13-22.

Caufield PW, Cutter GR, Dasanayake AP (1993). Initial acquisition of mutans streptococci by infants: evidence for a discrete window of infectivity. *J Dent Res* 72:37-45.

Diamanti J, Townsend GC (2003). New standards for permanent tooth emergence in Australian children. *Aust Dent J* 48:39-42.

Fraga MF, Ballestar E, Paz MF, Ropero S, Setien F, Ballestar ML, et al. (2005). Epigenetic differences arise during the lifetime of monozygotic twins. *Proc Natl Acad Sci U.S.A.* 102:10604-10609.

Geller F, Feenstra B, Zhang H, Shaffer JR, Hansen T, Esserlind A-L, et al. (2011). Genome-wide association study identifies four loci associated with eruption of permanent teeth. *PLoS Genet* 7:e1002275 doi:10.1371/journal.pgen.1002275. Accessed 19 May 2015.

Ha D, Roberts-Thomson K, Armfield J (2011). The Child Dental Health Surveys Australia, 2005 and 2006. *Dental statistics and research series no. 54. Cat. no. DEN 213*. Canberra: Australian Institute of Health and Welfare.

Hughes TE, Bockmann MR, Seow K, Gotjamanos T, Gully N, Richards LC, et al. (2007). Strong genetic control of emergence of human primary incisors. *J Dent Res* 86:1160-1165.

Hughes T, Townsend G (2013). Twin and family studies of human dental crown morphology: genetic, epigenetic, and environmental determinants of the modern human dentition. In: *Anthropological Perspectives on Tooth Morphology: genetics, evolution, variation.* Scott GR, Irish JD, editors. Cambridge: Cambridge University Press, pp. 31-68.

Hughes TE, Townsend GC, Pinkerton SK, Bockmann MR, Seow WK, Brook AH, et al. (2014). The teeth and faces of twins: providing insights into dentofacial development and oral health for practising health professionals. *Aust Dent J* 59 (1 Suppl):101-116.

Kaidonis J, Townsend G (2015). The 'Sialo-Microbial-Dental Complex' in oral health and disease. *Ann Anat.* doi:10.1016/j.aanat.2015.02.002. Accessed 19 May 2015.

Köhler B, Andréen I, Jonsson B (1988). The earlier the colonization by mutans streptococci, the higher the caries prevalence at 4 years of age. *Oral Microbiol Immunol* 3:14-17.

Liu F, van der Lijn F, Schurmann C, Zhu G, Chakravarty MM, Hysi PG, et al. (2012). A genome-wide association study identifies five loci influencing facial morphology in Europeans. *PLoS Genet* 8:e1002932 doi:10.1371/journal.pgen.1002932. Accessed 19 May 2015.

Mihailidis S, Woodroffe SN, Hughes TE, Bockmann MR, Townsend GC (2009). Patterns of asymmetry in primary tooth emergence of Australian twins. In: *Comparative Dental Morphology*. Koppe T, Meyer G, Alt KW, editors. Frontiers in Oral Biology, Basel: Karger, 2009, vol 13, pp. 110-115.

Miles CM, Wayne M (2008). Quantitative trait locus (QTL) analysis. *Scitable by Nature Education* 1:208. Accessed 30 July 2014.

Pillas D, Hoggart CJ, Evans DM, O'Reilly PF, Sipilä K, Lähdesmäki R, et al. (2010). Genome-wide association study reveals multiple loci associated with primary tooth development during infancy. *PLoS Genet* 6:e1000856 doi:10.1371/journal.pgen.1000856. Accessed 19 May 2015.

Stanley BO, Feingold E, Cooper M, Vanyukov MM, Maher BS, Slayton RL, et al. (2014). Genetic association of *MPPED2* and *ACTN2* with dental caries. *J Dent Res* 93:626-632.

Straetemans MM, van Loveren C, de Soet JJ, de Graaff J, ten Cate JM (1998). Colonization with mutans streptococci and lactobacilli and the caries experience of children after the age of five. *J Dent Res* 77:1851-1855.

Takahashi N, Nyvad B (2008). Caries ecology revisited: microbial dynamics and the caries process. *Caries Res* 42:409-418.

Townsend G, Bockmann M, Hughes T, Mihailidis S, Seow WK, Brook A (2012). New approaches to dental anthropology based on the study of twins. In: *New Directions in Dental Anthropology: paradigms, methodologies and outcomes*. Townsend G, Kanazawa E, Takayama H, editors. Adelaide: University of Adelaide Press, pp. 10-21.

Townsend GC, Brook AH (2014). The face, the future, and dental practice: how research in craniofacial biology will influence patient care. *Aust Dent J* 59 (1 Suppl):1-5.

Townsend G, Hughes T, Luciano M, Bockmann M, Brook A (2009). Genetic and environmental influences on human dental variation: a critical evaluation of studies involving twins. *Arch Oral Biol* 54S:S45-S51.

Waddington CH (1957). *The strategy of genes: a discussion of some aspects of theoretical biology.* London: Allen & Unwin.

Wan AKL, Seow WK, Purdie DM, Bird PS, Walsh LJ, Tudehope DI (2003). A longitudinal study of *Streptococcus mutans* colonization in infants after tooth eruption. *J Dent Res* 82:504-508.

Wan AKL, Seow WK, Walsh LJ, Bird P, Tudehope DI, Purdie DM (2001a). Association of *Streptococcus mutans* infection and oral development nodules in pre-dentate infants. *J Dent Res* 80:1945-1948.

Wan AKL, Seow WK, Purdie DM, Bird PS, Walsh LJ, Tudehope DI (2001b). Oral colonization of *Streptococcus mutans* in six-month-old predentate infants. *J Dent Res* 80:2060-2065.

Wang X, Shaffer JR, Weyant RJ, Cuenco KT, DeSensi RS, Crout R, et al. (2010). Genes and their effects on dental caries may differ between primary and permanent dentitions. *Caries Res* 44:277-284.

Williams SD, Hughes TE, Adler CJ, Brook AH, Townsend GC (2014). Epigenetics: a new frontier in dentistry. *Aust Dent J* 59 (1 Suppl):23-33.

Woodroffe S, Mihailidis S, Hughes T, Bockmann M, Seow K, Gotjamanos T, et al. (2010). Primary tooth emergence in Australian children: timing, sequence and patterns of asymmetry. *Aust Dent J* 55:245-251.

Yong R, Ranjitkar S, Townsend GC, Smith RN, Evans AR, Hughes TE, et al. (2014). Dental phenomics: advancing genotype to phenotype correlations in craniofacial research. *Aust Dent J* 59 (1 Suppl):34-47.

Chapter Seven

PUBLICATIONS AND THESES RELATING TO THE ADELAIDE TWIN STUDIES

PUBLICATIONS

1980s

Brown T, Townsend GC, Richards LC, Travan GR (1987). A study of dentofacial morphology in South Australian twins. *Aust Dent J* 32:81-90.

Sekikawa M, Namura T, Kanazawa E, Ozaki T, Richards LC, Townsend GC, Brown T (1989). Three-dimensional measurement of the maxillary first molar in Australian Whites. *Nihon Univ J Oral Sci* 15:457-464.

Townsend G (1988). Research in dentistry: growth and development. *Aust Dent J* 33:375-378.

Townsend GC, Corruccini RS, Richards LC, Brown T (1988). Genetic and environmental determinants of dental occlusion variation in South Australian twins. *Aust Orthod J* 10:231-235.

Townsend GC, Richards LC, Brown T, Burgess VB (1988). Twin zygosity determination on the basis of dental morphology. *J Forensic Odontostomatol* 6:1-15.

Townsend GC, Brown T, Richards LC, Rogers JR, Pinkerton SK, Travan GR, Burgess VB (1986). Metric analyses of the teeth and faces of South Australian twins. *Acta Genet Med Gemellol* 35:179-192.

Travan GR, Townsend GC, Brown T, Richards LC, Burgess VB (1987). Application of the SIR system in a study of South Australian twins. Proceedings of the Annual Conference USIR Australasia.

1990s

Brown T, Townsend GC, Richards LC, Travan GR, Pinkerton SK (1992). Facial symmetry and mirror imaging in South Australian twins. In: *Craniofacial Variation in Pacific Populations*. Brown T, Molnar S, editors. Adelaide: Anthropology and Genetics Laboratory, The University of Adelaide, pp. 79-98.

Corruccini RS, Townsend GC, Richards LC, Brown T (1990). Genetic and environmental determinants of dental occlusal variation in twins of different nationalities. *Hum Biol* 62:353-367.

Dempsey PJ, Townsend GC, Martin NG (1999). Insights into the genetic basis of human dental variation from statistical modelling analyses. *Perspec Hum Biol* 4(3):9-17.

Dempsey PJ, Townsend GC, Richards LC (1999). Increased tooth crown size in females with twin brothers: evidence for hormonal diffusion between human twins in utero. *Am J Hum Biol* 11:577-586.

Dempsey P, Schwerdt W, Townsend G, Richards L (1999). Handedness in twins: the search for genetic and environmental causes. *Perspec Hum Biol* 4(3):37-44.

Dempsey PJ, Townsend GC, Martin NG, Neale MC (1995). Genetic covariance structure of incisor crown size in twins. *J Dent Res* 74:1389-1398.

Kapali S, Townsend G, Richards L, Parish T (1997). Palatal rugae patterns in Australian Aborigines and Caucasians. *Aust Dent J* 42:129-133.

Kasai K, Richards LC, Townsend GC, Kanazawa E, Iwasawa T (1995). Fourier analysis of dental arch morphology in South Australian twins. *Anthropol Sci* 103:39-48.

Mealey L, Townsend GC (1999). The role of fluctuating asymmetry on judgements of physical attractiveness: a monozygotic co-twin comparison. *Perspec Hum Biol* 4(1):219-224.

Mealey L, Bridgstock R, Townsend GC (1998). Symmetry and perceived facial attractiveness: a monozygotic co-twin comparison. *J Pers Soc Psychol* 76:151-158.

Pinkerton S, Townsend G, Richards L, Schwerdt W, Dempsey P (1999). Expression of Carabelli trait in both dentitions of Australian twins. *Perspec Hum Biol* 4(3):19-28.

Richards LC, Townsend GC, Brown T, Burgess VB (1990). Dental arch morphology in South Australian twins. *Arch Oral Biol* 35:983-989.

Richards LC, Townsend GC, Kasai K (1997). Application of the Fourier method on genetic studies of dentofacial morphology. In: *Fourier Descriptors and their Application in Biology.* Lestrel PE, editor. Cambridge: Cambridge University Press, pp. 189-209.

Springbett SM, Townsend GC, Kaidonis J, Richards LC (1999). Tooth wear in the deciduous dentition: a cross-cultural and longitudinal study. *Perspec Hum Biol* 4(3):93-101.

Thomas CJ, Townsend GC (1999). Anterior spacing in the primary dentition: a study of Australian twins and singletons. *Perspec Hum Biol* 4(3):29-35.

Townsend GC (1992). Genetic and environmental contributions to morphometric dental variation. In: *Culture, Ecology and Dental Anthropology.* Lukacs JR, editor. Delhi: Kamla-Raj, pp. 61-72.

Townsend G (1994). Understanding the nature and causes of variation in dento-facial structures. *Proc Finn Dent Soc* 12:642-648.

Townsend G, Richards L (1990). Twins and twinning, dentists and dentistry. *Aust Dent J* 35:317-327.

Townsend GC, Martin NG (1992). Fitting genetic models to Carabelli trait data in South Australian twins. *J Dent Res* 71:403-409.

Townsend GC, Richards LC, Brown T (1992). Mirror imaging in the dentitions of twins — what is the biological basis? In: *Craniofacial Variation in Pacific Populations.* Brown T, Molnar S, editors. Adelaide: Anthropology and Genetics Laboratory, The University of Adelaide, pp. 67-78.

Townsend GC, Aldred MJ, Bartold PM (1998). Genetic aspects of dental disorders. *Aust Dent J* 43:269-286.

Townsend G, Dempsey P, Richards L (1999). Asymmetry in the deciduous dentition: fluctuating and directional components. *Perspec Hum Biol* 4(3):45-52.

Townsend G, Dempsey P, Richards L (1999). Causal components of dental variation: new approaches using twins. In: *Dental Morphology 1998: Proceedings of 11th International Symposium on Dental Morphology*. Mayhall JT, Heikkinen T, editors. Oulu: University of Oulu Press, pp. 464-472.

Townsend G, Richards L, Brown T, Pinkerton S (1994). Mirror imaging in twins: some dental examples. *Dent Anthropol Newsl* 9:2-5.

Townsend G, Rogers J, Richards L, Brown T (1995). Agenesis of permanent maxillary lateral incisors in South Australian twins. *Aust Dent J* 40:186-192.

Townsend GC, Richards LC, Sekikawa M, Brown T, Ozaki T (1990). Variability of palatal dimensions in South Australian twins. *J Forensic Odontostomatol* 8:3-14.

Townsend G, Dempsey P, Brown T, Kaidonis J, Richards L (1994). Teeth, genes and the environment. *Perspec Hum Biol* 4:35-46.

Townsend GC, Richards LC, Brown T, Burgess VB, Travan GR, Rogers JR (1992). Genetic studies of dental morphology in South Australian twins. In: *Structure, Function and Evolution of Teeth*. Smith P, Tchernov E, editors. London: Freund Publishing House, pp. 501-518.

Vanco C, Kasai K, Sergi R, Richards LC, Townsend GC (1995). Genetic and environmental influences on facial profile. *Aust Dent J* 40:104-109.

2000s

Apps MV, Hughes TE, Townsend GC (2004). The effect of birthweight on tooth-size variability in twins. *Twin Res* 7:415-420.

Chegini-Farahini S, Fuss J, Townsend G (2000). Intra- and inter-population variability in mamelon expression on incisor teeth. *Dent Anthropol* 14:1-6.

Corruccini RS, Townsend GC (2003). Decline in enamel hypoplasia in relation to fluoridation in Australians. *Am J Hum Biol* 15:795-799.

Corruccini RS, Townsend GC, Schwerdt W (2005). Correspondence between enamel hypoplasia and odontometric bilateral asymmetry in Australian twins. *Am J Phys Anthropol* 126:177-182.

Darwis WE, Messer LB, Thomas CDL (2003). Assessing growth and development of the facial profile. *Pediatr Dent* 25:103-108.

Dempsey PJ, Townsend GC (2001). Genetic and environmental contributions to variation in human tooth size. *Heredity* 86:685-693.

Dooland KV, Townsend GC, Kaidonis JA (2006). Prevalence and side preference for tooth grinding in twins. *Aust Dent J* 51:219-224.

Eguchi S, Townsend GC, Richards LC, Hughes T, Kasai K (2004). Genetic contribution to dental arch size variation in Australian twins. *Arch Oral Biol* 49:1015-1024.

Eguchi S, Townsend GC, Hughes T, Kasai K (2004). Genetic and environmental contributions to variation in the inclination of human mandibular molars. *Orthod Waves* 63:95-100.

Higgins D, Hughes TE, James H, Townsend GC (2009). Strong genetic influence on hypocone expression of permanent maxillary molars in South Australian twins. *Dent Anthropol* 22:1-7.

Hughes T, Richards L, Townsend G (2001). Dental arch form in young Australian twins. In: *Dental Morphology 2001*. Brook A, editor. Sheffield, England: Sheffield Academic Press, pp. 309-319.

Hughes T, Richards L, Townsend G (2002). Form, symmetry and asymmetry of the dental arch: orthogonal analysis revisited. *Dent Anthropol* 16:3-8.

Hughes T, Thomas C, Richards L, Townsend G (2001). A study of occlusal variation in the primary dentition of Australian twins and singletons. *Arch Oral Biol* 46:857-864.

Hughes T, Dempsey P, Richards L, Townsend G (2000). Genetic analysis of deciduous tooth size in Australian twins. *Arch Oral Biol* 45:997-1004.

Hughes TE, Bockmann MR, Seow K, Gotjamanos T, Gully N, Richards LC, Townsend GC (2007). Strong genetic control of emergence of human primary incisors. *J Dent Res* 86:1160-1165.

Kondo S, Townsend GC (2006). Associations between Carabelli trait and cusp areas in human permanent maxillary first molars. *Am J Phys Anthropol* 129:196-203.

Kondo S, Townsend GC, Yamada H (2005). Sexual dimorphism of cusp dimensions in human maxillary molars. *Am J Phys Anthropol* 128:870-877.

Liu P, Ranjitkar S, Kaidonis JA, Townsend GC, Richards LC (2004). A system for the acquisition and analysis of three-dimensional data describing dental morphology. *Dent Anthropol* 17:70-74.

Medland SE, Duffy DL, Wright MJ, Geffen G, Hay DA, Levyl F, Catherina EM, van-Beijsterveldt CEM, Willemsen G, Townsend GC, White V, Hewitt AW, Mackey DA, Bailey JM,. Slutske WS, Nyholta DR, Treloar SA, Martin NG, Boomsma DI (2009). Genetic influences on handedness: data from 25 732 Australian and Dutch twin families. *Neuropsychologia* 47:330-337.

Mihailidis S, Woodroffe SN, Hughes TE, Bockmann MR, Townsend G (2009). Patterns of asymmetry in primary tooth emergence of Australian twins. In: *Comparative Dental Morphology*. Koppe T, Meyer G, Alt KW, editors. Frontiers in Oral Biology, Basel: Karger, 2009, vol 13, pp. 110-115.

Race JP, Townsend GC, Hughes TE (2006). Chorion type, birth weight discordance and tooth-size variability in Australian monozygotic twins. *Twin Res Hum Genet* 9:285-291.

Smith RN, Townsend G, Chen K, Brook A (2009). Synetic superimposition of dental 3D data: application in twin studies. In: *Comparative Dental Morphology*. Koppe T, Meyer G, Alt KW, editors. Frontiers in Oral Biology, Basel: Karger, 2009, vol 13, pp. 142-147.

Smith R, Zaitoun H, Coxon T, Karmo M, Kaur G, Townsend G, Harris EF, Brook A (2009). Defining new dental phenotypes using 3-D image analysis to enhance discrimination and insights into biological processes. *Arch Oral Biol* 54S:S118-S125.

Taji S, Hughes T, Rogers J, Townsend G (2000). Localised enamel hypoplasia of human deciduous canines: genotype or environment? *Aust Dent J* 45:83-90.

Takahashi M, Kondo S, Townsend GC, Kanazawa E (2007). Variability in cusp size of human maxillary molars, with particular reference to the hypocone. *Arch Oral Biol* 52:1146-1154.

Tangchaitrong K, Messer LB, Thomas CDL, Townsend GC (2000). Fourier analysis of facial profiles of young twins. *Am J Phys Anthropol* 113:369-379.

Townsend G (2006). Comparing 'identical' twin pairs — a research model for busy clinicians. *Dental Insights* 19:11-13.

Townsend G, Brook A (2008). Genetic, epigenetic and environmental influences on the human dentition. *Ortho Tribune* 3:3-6.

Townsend G, Alvesalo L, Brook A (2008). Variation in the human dentition: some past advances and future opportunities. *J Dent Res* 87:802-805.

Townsend GC, Hughes T, Richards L (2005). The dentitions of monozygotic twin pairs: focussing on the differences rather than the similarities. In: *Current Trends in Dental Morphology Research*. Refereed full papers, 13th International Symposium on Dental Morphology. Zadzinska E, editor. Poland: University of Lodz, pp. 337-352.

Townsend G, Hughes T, Richards LC (2006). Gaining new insights into how genetic factors influence human dental development by studying twins. *Int J Anthropol* 21:67-74.

Townsend G, Richards L, Hughes T (2003). Molar intercuspal dimensions: genetic input to phenotypic variation. *J Dent Res* 82:350-355.

Townsend G, Harris EF, Lesot H, Clauss F, Brook A (2009). Morphogenetic fields within the human dentition: a new, clinically relevant synthesis of an old concept. *Arch Oral Biol* 54S:S34-S44.

Townsend G, Hughes T, Bockmann M, Smith R, Brook A (2009). How studies of twins can inform our understanding of dental morphology. In: *Comparative Dental Morphology*. Koppe T, Meyer G, Alt KW, editors. Frontiers in Oral Biology, Basel: Karger, 2009, vol 13, pp. 136-141.

Townsend G, Hughes T, Luciano M, Bockmann M, Brook A (2009). Genetic and environmental influences on human dental variation: a critical evaluation of studies involving twins. *Arch Oral Biol* 54S:S45-S51.

Townsend GC, Richards L, Hughes T, Pinkerton S, Schwerdt W (2003). The value of twins in dental research. *Aust Dent J* 48:82-88.

Townsend GC, Richards L, Hughes T, Pinkerton S, Schwerdt W (2005). Epigenetic influences may explain dental differences in monozygotic twin pairs. *Aust Dent J* 50:95-100.

Townsend G, Richards L, Messer LB, Hughes T, Pinkerton S, Seow K, Gotjamanos T, Gully N, Bockmann M (2006). Genetic and environmental influences on dentofacial structures and oral health: studies of Australian twins and their families. *Twin Res Hum Genet* 9:727-732.

2010 TO 2015

Ashar A, Hughes T, James H, Kaidonis J, Khamis F, Townsend G (2012). Dental crown and arch size in Europeans and Australian Aboriginals In: *New Directions in Dental Anthropology: paradigms, methodologies and outcomes.* Townsend G, Kanazawa E, Takayama H, editors. Adelaide: University of Adelaide Press, pp. 65-80.

Bockmann MR, Hughes TE, Townsend GC (2010). Genetic modeling of primary tooth emergence: a study of Australian twins. *Twin Res Hum Genet* 13:573-581.

Bockmann MR, Harris AV, Bennett CN, Odeh R, Hughes TE, Townsend GC (2011). Timing of colonization of caries-producing bacteria: an approach based on studying monozygotic twin pairs. *Int J Dent*, Article ID 571573, 7 pages, doi:10.1155/2011/571573. Accessed 19 May 2015.

Chan E, Bockmann M, Hughes T, Mihailidis S, Townsend G (2012). Do feeding practices, gestation length, and birth weight affect the timing of emergence of the first primary tooth? In: *New Directions in Dental Anthropology: paradigms, methodologies and outcomes.* Townsend G, Kanazawa E, Takayama H, editors. Adelaide: University of Adelaide Press, pp. 35-45.

Hasegawa Y, Rogers J, Scriven G, Townsend G (2010). Carabelli trait in Australian twins: reliability and validity of different scoring systems. *Dent Anthropol* 23:7-14.

Hughes T, Townsend G (2012). Genes for teeth — drawing inference from family data. In: *New Directions in Dental Anthropology: paradigms, methodologies and outcomes.* Townsend G, Kanazawa E, Takayama H, editors. Adelaide: University of Adelaide Press, pp. 22-34.

Hughes T, Bockmann M, Mihailidis S, Bennett C, Harris A, Seow WK, Lekkas D, Ranjitkar S, Rupinskas L, Pinkerton S, Brook A, Smith R, Townsend GC (2013). Genetic, epigenetic, and environmental influences on dentofacial structures and oral health: ongoing studies of Australian twins and their families. *Twin Res Hum Genet* 16:43-51.

Hughes TE, Townsend GC (2013). Twin and family studies of human dental crown morphology: genetic, epigenetic and environmental determinants of the modern human dentition. In: *Anthropological Perspectives on Tooth Morphology: genetics, evolution, variation.* Scott GR, Irish JD, editors. Cambridge: Cambridge University Press, pp. 31-68.

Hughes TE, Townsend GC, Pinkerton SK, Bockmann MR, Seow Wk, Brook AH, Richards LC, Mihailidis S, Ranjitkar S, Lekkas D (2014). The teeth and faces of twins: providing insights into dentofacial development and oral health for practicing oral health professionals. *Aust Dent J* 59 (1 Suppl):101-116.

Hughes T, Bockmann M, Townsend G (2015). An overview of dental genetics. In: *A Companion to Dental Anthropology.* Irish JD, Scott GR, editors. Hoboken, NJ: John Wiley & Sons Inc. (in press).

Kondo S, Townsend G, Matsuno M (2014). Morphological variation of the maxillary lateral incisor. *Jpn Dent Sci Rev* 50:100-107.

Mihailidis S, Scriven G, Khamis M, Townsend G (2013). Prevalence and patterning of maxillary premolar accessory ridges (MxPARs) in several human populations. *Am J Phys Anthropol* 152:19-30.

Mihailidis S, Ashar A, Hughes T, Bockmann M, Brook A, Townsend G (2013). Dental phenomics: high-tech scans reveal similarities and differences in monozygotic twins. *Dental Tribune US Edition* April:A4-A5.

Mihailidis S, Bockmann M, McConnell E, Hughes T, van Beijsterveldt TCEM, Boomsma DI, McMaster M, Townsend G (2015). The influence of chorion type on health measures at birth and dental development in Australian and Dutch twins: a comparative study. *Twin Res Hum Genet* 18:368-374.

Odeh R, Mihailidis S, Townsend G, Lähdesmäki R, Hughes T, Brook A (2015). Prevalence of infraocclusion of primary molars determined using a new 2D image analysis methodology. *Aust Dent J* (in press).

Odeh R, Townsend G, Mihailidis S, Lähdesmäki R, Hughes T, Brook A (2015). Infraocclusion: dental development and associated dental variations in singleton and twins. *Arch Oral Biol* 60:1394-1402.

Ooi G, Townsend G, Seow WK (2014). Bacterial colonization, enamel defects and dental caries in 4-6-year-old mono- and dizygotic twins. *Int J Paediatr Dent* 24:152-160.

Ribeiro DC, Brook AH, Hughes TE, Sampson WJ, Townsend GC (2013). Intrauterine hormone effects on tooth dimensions. *J Dent Res* 92:425-431.

Ribeiro D, Sampson W, Hughes T, Brook A, Townsend G (2012). Sexual dimorphism in the primary and permanent dentitions of twins: an approach to clarifying the role of hormonal factors. In: *New Directions in Dental Anthropology: paradigms, methodologies and outcomes.* Townsend G, Kanazawa E, Takayama H, editors. Adelaide: University of Adelaide Press, pp. 46-64.

Taji SS, Seow WK, Townsend GC, Holcombe T (2010). A controlled study of dental erosion in 2- to 4-year-old twins. *Int J Paediatr Dent* 20:400-409.

Taji SS, Seow WK, Townsend GC, Holcombe T (2011). Enamel hypoplasia in the primary dentition of monozygous and dizygous twins compared with singleton controls. *Int J Paediatr Dent* 21:175-184.

Townsend GC, Brook AH (2013). Genetic, epigenetic and environmental influences on human tooth size, shape and number. In: *eLS*. Chichester: John Wiley & Sons, Ltd. doi:10.1002/9780470015902.a0024858. Accessed 19 May 2015.

Townsend GC, Brook AH (2014). The face, the future, and dental practice: how research in craniofacial biology will influence patient care. *Aust Dent J* 59 (1 Suppl):1-5.

Townsend G, Bockmann M, Hughes T, Brook A (2012). Genetic, environmental and epigenetic influences on variation in human tooth number, size and shape. *Odontology* 100:1-9.

Townsend G, Bockmann M, Hughes T, Mihailidis S, Seow WK, Brook A (2012). New approaches to dental anthropology based on the study of twins. In: *New Directions in Dental Anthropology: paradigms, methodologies and outcomes.* Townsend G, Kanazawa E, Takayama H, editors. Adelaide: University of Adelaide Press, pp. 10-21.

Townsend G, Brook A, Yong R, Hughes T (2015). Tooth classes, field concepts, and symmetry. In: *A Companion to Dental Anthropology.* Irish JD, Scott GR, editors. Hoboken, NJ: John Wiley & Sons Inc. (in press).

Woodroffe S, Mihailidis S, Hughes T, Bockmann M, Seow WK, Gotjamanos T, Townsend G (2010). Primary tooth emergence in Australian children: timing, sequence and patterns of asymmetry. *Aust Dent J* 55:245-251.

Yong R, Ranjitkar S, Townsend GC, Smith RN, Evans AR, Hughes TE, Lekkas D, Brook AH (2014). Dental phenomics: advancing genotype to phenotype correlations in craniofacial research. *Aust Dent J* 59 (1 Suppl):34-47.

Theses

Richmond D (1990). *An assessment of dental occlusion in a sample of South Australian twins.* BScDent (Hons) Thesis, The University of Adelaide.

Rogers JR (1990). *Tooth size variability in South Australian twins.* BScDent (Hons) Thesis, The University of Adelaide.

Townsend GC (1994). *Genetic studies of morphological variation in the human dentition.* DDSc Thesis, The University of Adelaide.

Dempsey P (1998). *Genetic and environmental contributions to morphological variation in the permanent dentition — a study of Australian twins.* PhD Thesis, The University of Adelaide.

Tangchaitrong K (1998). *Fourier shape analysis of facial profiles of twins.* MDS Thesis, The University of Melbourne.

Thomas C (1998). *Occlusal variation in the primary dentition: a study of Australian twins and singletons.* MDS Thesis, The University of Adelaide.

Chegini-Farahani A (1999). *Incisor mamelon morphology: how important are genetic factors.* BScDent (Hons) Thesis, The University of Adelaide.

Darwis WE (2002). *Fourier analysis: assessment of facial profile variation with time in young twins.* MDS Thesis, The University of Melbourne.

Loo SM (2003). *Growth of facial features in young twins: assessment by Fourier shape analysis.* MDS Thesis, The University of Melbourne.

Chiam S (2004). *Superimposition of computer-generated overlays of anterior teeth in pairs of identical twins.* Grad Dip Forensic Odont Thesis, The University of Adelaide.

Apps M (2005). *Effect of birthweight on tooth size variability in twins.* BScDent (Hons) Thesis, The University of Adelaide.

Dooland K (2005). *Is there a side preference for bruxing?* BScDent (Hons) Thesis, The University of Adelaide.

Race J (2005). *Birthweight discordance and chorion type in monozygotic twins.* BScDent (Hons) Thesis, The University of Adelaide.

Ramadas Y (2005). *Longitudinal studies of facial growth of twins.* DClinDent Thesis. The University of Melbourne.

Mahmood Z (2006). *Age changes in dental arch shape in twins.* MDS Thesis, The University of Adelaide.

Ismail Z (2006). *Hypocone expression in Australian twins.* Grad Dip Forensic Odont Thesis, The University of Adelaide.

Woodroffe S (2006). *Factors influencing tooth emergence in young twins.* BScDent (Hons) Thesis, The University of Adelaide.

Odeh R (2008). *Mutans streptococci and their relationship with primary tooth emergence.* BScDent (Hons) Thesis, The University of Adelaide.

Smythe L (2008). *Identification of individuals by superimposition of dental structures.* Grad Dip Forensic Odont Thesis, The University of Adelaide.

Taji S (2010). *A controlled study of oral health in twin children.* DClinDent Thesis, The University of Queensland.

Bermann H (2011). *Variation in human palatal rugae and their use as a forensic marker.* BScDent (Hons) Thesis, The University of Adelaide.

Chan E (2011). *Effect of feeding habits on primary tooth emergence.* BScDent (Hons) Thesis, The University of Adelaide.

Handayani A (2011). *Validation of an Optix 400S 3D laser scanner for use in forensic odontology.* Grad Dip Forensic Odont Thesis, The University of Adelaide.

McConnell E (2011). *The influence of chorion type on the emergence of first primary tooth in Australian twins.* BScDent (Hons) Thesis, The University of Adelaide.

Ribeiro D (2012). *Increased tooth crown size in females from opposite-sex dizygotic twins: a possible intrauterine hormonal influence on dental development.* PhD Thesis, The University of Adelaide.

Williams S (2012). *Epigenetic influences on dental development.* BScDent (Hons) Thesis, The University of Adelaide.

Bullens L (2013). *Evidence of tooth grinding patterns in twins — side preference, mirror-imaging and handedness.* Masters Thesis, Academisch Centrum Tandhellkunde Amsterdam.

Publications and theses relating to the Adelaide Twin Studies

Cheshire K (2013). *Tooth grinding in the primary and permanent dentitions of twins.* Masters Thesis, Academisch Centrum Tandhellkunde Amsterdam.

Gagliardi A (2013). *A genetic analysis of the Curve of Spee.* DClinDent Thesis, The University of Adelaide.

Odeh R (2013). *Infraocclusion of primary molars and associated dental anomalies in twins and singletons: what is the underlying aetiology.* PhD Thesis, The University of Adelaide.

Ashar A (2015). *The individuality of the human dentition: implications for forensic odontology.* PhD Thesis, The University of Adelaide.

Patel P (2015). *Intrauterine male hormone effects on dental dimensions of females from dizygotic opposite-sex twin pairs.* BScDent (Hons) Thesis, The University of Adelaide.

Lam F (ongoing). *Exploring further the different effects of the Y chromosome and male hormones on tooth size and shape by 3D measurement and analysis on twin study models.* BScDent (Hons) Thesis, The University of Adelaide.

Taduran RJ (ongoing). *The nature and extent of sexual dimorphism in dental and dermatoglyphic traits of twins.* PhD Thesis, The University of Adelaide.

Williams S (ongoing). *Epigenetic studies of dental development and the oral microbiome.* PhD Thesis, The University of Sydney.

Waller D (ongoing). *Sequence of primary tooth emergence in twins.* BScDent (Hons) Thesis, The University of Adelaide.

Ribeiro D (ongoing). *Development of dental occlusion and speech in Australian twins.* DClinDent Thesis, The University of Adelaide.

GLOSSARY OF TERMS

Acetylation — The process or formation of an acetyl (an acetic acid molecule) derivative. Acetylation of histone proteins reduces the affinity between these proteins and DNA in the nucleus of the cell and is another epigenetic mechanism (in addition to methylation) to control gene expression.

Aetiology — The cause or set of causes of a disease or disorder.

Agenesis — Absence or failure of a structure to develop, e.g. a tooth.

Algorithm — A process or set of rules used in problem-solving calculations and operations.

Amniotic — Relating to the amnion, a membrane that envelops the embryo in utero.

Androgens — Androgens (which include testosterone) are often referred to as 'male hormones', although males and females both produce androgens. They are present in higher levels in males and play an important role in male traits and reproductive activity.

Anthropometric — Related to measurements of the human body.

Biofilm (oral) — A thin coating that contains bacteria and forms over structures in the mouth, e.g. teeth.

Buccal — Relating to the cheeks.

Buccolingual crown diameter — The distance between the buccal (cheek) and lingual (tongue) surfaces of a dental crown. For anterior teeth, the term 'labiolingual' is often used, where 'labial' refers to the lips.

Glossary of terms

Cariogenic — Producing dental decay.

Cerebral lateralisation — Refers to specialisation of the two halves of the brain, with one side carrying out certain functions and the other side performing different functions. For example, the right side has been linked to language production and the left side to visuo-spatial perception.

Chi-square test — Statistical test whereby variables are categorised to determine whether an observed distribution of scores differs from those expected according to a certain hypothesis.

Chorion — One of the foetal membranes.

Chromosome — One of the rod-shaped structures situated in the nucleus of a cell that carries genes. There are usually 22 pairs of autosomes (numbered 1 to 22) and one pair of sex chromosomes (X and Y) in humans, making 23 pairs or 46 chromosomes in total.

Cohort — A collection of people sharing similar characteristics.

Congenital — Refers to conditions which are present at birth and may be either hereditary or due to an influence occurring during gestation.

Correlation coefficient — A statistical measure of the strength of the association between two variables, often denoted by the symbol r. Values can range from -1 to +1 with a value of 0 indicating no association.

Covariance — Statistical measure of how much two variables change together.

Deciduous (primary) — Teeth that are shed (exfoliated) and replaced by permanent teeth.

Dental caries — The process involving loss of mineral from the teeth due to acid production by bacteria within dental plaque (oral biofilm).

Dental lamina — A curved band of epithelium in the upper and lower developing jaws with growths (or swellings) at the sites where future deciduous teeth will form.

Dental papilla(e) — Clump(s) of mesenchymal cells which give rise to the dentine and pulp of the teeth. Neural crest cells contribute to the dental papilla, so the cells are often referred to as ecto-mesenchymal, referring to the ectodermal origin of the neural crest.

Dermatoglyphics	The study of fingerprints.
Dichorionic	Showing evidence of two chorions (foetal membranes) which enclose the foetus. Some monozygotic (so-called identical) twin pairs are dichorionic, whereas others are monochorionic.
Digitiser	Equipment that has the ability to locate features on images or models and convert the data generated into a digital format for storage on a computer.
Ectoderm	The outer layer of cells in an embryo.
Enamel organ	Refers to the epithelially derived component of the developing tooth germ which eventually forms the enamel of the crown.
Endoderm	The innermost of the three primary layers of cells in an embryo.
Epidemiology	The study of the patterns, causes and outcomes of conditions affecting health and disease in human populations.
Epigenetics	Refers to the regulation of gene expression without changing the genetic code.
Ethnicity	Related to a group of people who share a distinctive social and cultural tradition, often established by their origin at birth.
Eugenics	The study of, or the belief in, improving the genetic quality of human populations. There have been attempts at both 'positive eugenics' (by selective breeding of those with 'desirable' features), and 'negative eugenics' (by eliminating those with 'undesirable' features).
Exfoliation	The normal process of loss of deciduous (primary) teeth, which occurs as their roots are resorbed.
Extrinsic	Coming from outside, e.g. extrinsic factors coming from outside the body, such as trauma, may damage tooth structure.
Genome	The complete set of genes which constitute an organism.
Genotype	The genetic constitution of an individual.
Gingivitis	Inflammation of gingival tissue as a response to products of bacteria in dental plaque around the necks of teeth.
Homeostasis	The process through which bodily equilibrium is maintained.
Homologous	Corresponding or similar in position, structure or function, e.g. homologous chromosomes form pairs.

Glossary of terms

Hydroxyapatite	Natural mineral structure which is the principal inorganic component of bones and teeth.
Hypodontia	A congenital or acquired condition where there is less than the normal complement of teeth.
Hypoplasia	Condition illustrating defective or incomplete tissue. Enamel hypoplasia refers to a condition where the enamel of teeth is thinner than normal. It may present as linear grooves or pits on the tooth surface.
Hypothesis	A proposed explanation which is either retained or rejected depending on the outcomes of testing.
In utero	Within the womb.
Intercorrelated variables	Variables showing a mutual relationship or association.
Internal enamel epithelium	An epithelial layer in the developing tooth germ which folds to produce the basic shape of the future dental crown. The epithelial cells differentiate into ameloblasts that lay down enamel.
Intra-uterine	Within the womb.
Intrinsic	Coming from inside, e.g. intrinsic factors, such as proteins produced by the body.
Locus (plural is *loci*)	A particular position, point, place or location. In genetics, a locus refers to the specific location of a gene or DNA sequence on a chromosome.
Lupus erythematosus	A chronic inflammatory autoimmune disease that can affect various parts of the body, including the skin and joints.
Malocclusion	Term used to describe a variation from the 'ideal' or 'normal' relationship of the upper and lower teeth, e.g. crooked teeth, protruding 'buck' teeth.
Milieu intérieur	The environment within (French).
Mesenchyme	Embryonic connective tissue consisting of cells, fibres and ground substance.
Mesial surface	The surface of a tooth nearest to the midline of the dental arch.

Mesiodistal crown diameter	The distance between the mesial (nearest to the midline) and distal (furthest from the midline) surfaces of a dental crown.
Mesoderm	The middle layer of cells in an embryo.
Methylation	Addition of a methyl group, e.g. DNA methylation is one of the epigenetic mechanisms cells use to control the expression of genes.
Microbiome (oral)	The aggregate or community of micro-organisms found in the oral cavity.
Microbiota	A collective term for all of the micro-organisms found within a given environment.
Mirror imaging	Two images or structures, with one being the reverse of the other (as if seen in a mirror).
Modularity	The arrangement of a system into discrete units.
Monochorionic	Evidence of one chorion (also see dichorionic).
Morphogenesis	The development of a distinct shape during embryological development.
Morphology	The study of the form of living organisms.
Multiparous	Giving birth to more than one offspring at a time.
Multivariate analysis	Statistical term used for analyses involving more than one variable at a time.
Neural crest cells	Ectodermal cells derived from the developing neural tube. These cells have the potential to develop into a variety of tissues, including all of the tissues of teeth, except for the enamel.
Occlusion (dental)	Simply, dental occlusion refers to the contact between maxillary and mandibular teeth. More broadly, it refers to understanding of the structure and function of the masticatory system and managing problems within this system. In this sense, occlusion is basic to dentistry.
Odontogenesis	Tooth formation.
Odontometrics	The measurement and study of tooth size.
Orthopantomogram (OPG)	A panoramic radiograph used to provide an image of all of the teeth and the surrounding oral and facial structures.

Glossary of terms

PCR (Polymerase Chain Reaction) amplicons	The multiple segments of DNA replicated from a template during a Polymerase Chain Reaction process for amplifying DNA material.
Pergamon	Ancient city situated in Aeolis, an area once established along the north-western coastline of Asia Minor.
Periodontal disease	An inflammatory disease of the gingival tissues (gums) and supporting structures (periodontium) of teeth associated with the production of bacterial products from dental plaque around the necks of the teeth. This disease leads to loss of bone around the roots of teeth (alveolar bone) and to loosening (mobility) of the teeth.
Phenomics	The measurement of 'phenomes' that are usually associated with the physical and biochemical traits of organisms. Dental phenomics refers to measurement of variables of interest in dentistry, e.g. tooth size.
Phenotypes	Those observable characteristics of an individual which have been shaped from genetic, epigenetic and environmental influences.
Phylogenetics	Studies of evolutionary relationships among groups of organisms or populations.
Pleiotrophy	A situation where a gene appears to affect multiple features or traits.
Polyembryony	Development of more than one embryo from a fertilised egg.
Polygenic	Referring to more than one gene affecting a character or trait.
Sexual dimorphism	The difference in expression of a feature between males and females of the same species, e.g. males have larger teeth, on average, than females.
Sine/cosine	Mathematical function concerning angles.
Standard dental plaques	Standardised models that illustrate different expressions of dental traits to facilitate scoring of the features, e.g. the Arizona State University (ASU) plaques and the Dahlberg plaques.

Stereophoto-grammetry	A method of identifying landmarks and making measurements from two photographs taken from known positions in relation to the object of interest, e.g. a person's face.
Stochastic process	Random process.
Streptococcus mutans	Cariogenic (decay-producing) bacteria commonly found in dental plaque. The term *Streptococcus mutans* is used to refer to a single species of bacteria whereas the term mutans streptococci refers to a group of the streptococcal species.
Syndrome	A group of signs and symptoms that consistently occur together.
Systemic	Relating to, or affecting, the body as a whole, as distinct from a 'local' effect or disease.
Teratology	The study of abnormalities of development.
Variable	Feature being studied that can take on different values.
Vedic	The period and religion associated with ancient Indo-European speaking people who migrated to India from 1500 BC.
Zygosity	Refers to the degree of identity in the genome of twins. Monozygotic twins share the same genes, whereas dizygotic twins share, on average, half their genes.

APPENDIX 1

THE ORIGINAL RESEARCH TEAM

Grant Townsend
Lindsay Richards
Tasman Brown
Sandy Pinkerton
George Travan

CRANIOFACIAL BIOLOGY AND DENTAL EDUCATION GROUP 2015

Abdulaziz Almajed	Frances Greenwood	Caroline Petroff
Poppy Anastassiadis	Linda Hassanali	Renée Phillips
Peter Anderson	Toby Hughes	Sandy Pinkerton
Nor Atika Md Ashar	Helen James	Rabiah Rahmat
Manpreet Bariana	John Kaidonis	Sarbin Ranjitkar
Corinna Bennett	Sophie Karanicolas	Chris Redwood
John Berketa	Kenneth Koh	Daniela Ribeiro
Vishesh Bhojwani	Felicity Lam	James Rogers
Michelle Bockmann	Dimitra Lekkas	Ruth Rogers
Alan Brook	Chelsea Mann	Graham Scriven
Tasman Brown	Mustafa Mian	Komal Shah
Ketki Chandewar	Suzanna Mihailidis	Catherine Sims
Anh Diep	Ruba Odeh	Vicki Skinner
Mohamed El-Kishawi	Premal Patel	Catherine Snelling

Karen Squires
Richard Jonathan Taduran
Vivian Toh
Ikuko Tomo
Soichiro Tomo

Grant Townsend
Ryuji Ueno
Daniel Waller
Abbe White
Tom Wilkinson

Scott Williams
Tracey Winning
Robin Yong

Visiting researchers, collaborators and other key contributors

Wadian Abdul-Wahed
Hiro Aboshi
Christina Adler
Michael Aldred
Lassi Alvesalo
Mary Apps
Peter Arrow
Mark Bartold
Hannah Berman
Jasmine Blight
Lucas Bockmann
Dorret Boomsma
Louise Brearley Messer
Walter Bretz
Gary Briscoe
Bridget Brown
Gina Browne
Lotte Bullens
Viv Burgess
Hanny Calache
Angus Cameron
Emmanuel Chan
Ke Chen
Rebecca Chen
Kitty Cheshire
David Chubb
John Clement
Deborah Cole
Robert Corruccini

Tom Coxon
Jeffrey Craig
Paula Dempsey
John Diamanti
Kim Dooland
Craig Dreyer
Shosei Eguchi
Tennent Emerson
Alistair Evans
Luca Fiorenza
Judy Ford
Antonio Gagliardi
Jinlong Gao
Rakesh Garayia
Evangeline Gotjamanos
Theo Gotjamanos
Neville Gully
Edward Harris
Yuh Hasegawa
Shirley Hastings
David Hay
Tuomo Heikkinen
Denice Higgins
Jenny Hong
John Hopper
Neil Hunter
Tadashi Ideguchi
Elka Johansson
Ikuo Kageyama

Voula Kaidonis
Eisaku Kanazawa
Sunita Kapali
Kazutaka Kasai
Samvit Kaul
Mohd Fadhli Bin Khamis
Nima Kianoush
John Kibble
Jules Kieser
Nicky Kilpatrick
Inger Kjaer
Shintaro Kondo
Raija Lähdesmäki
Herve Lesot
Judith Littleton
Helen Liversidge
Pamela Long
Michelle Luciano
Lucy Ludlow
David Madsen
Zuliani Mahmood
Nick Martin
Judith May
John Mayhall
Elise McConnell
Linda Mealey
Sarah Medland
Pascale Mehanna
Marion Morgenstern

Appendix 1

John Mulley	Fiona Rowett	Kanokwan Tangchaitrong
Sen Nakahara	Loreta Rupinskas	Lydia Tarnowskyj
Koh Nakajima	Richard Saffery	Peter Telfer
Mike Neale	Wayne Sampson	Candy Thomas
Leanne Ng	Bhim Savara	David Thomas
Ruba Odeh	Wendy Schwerdt	Maureen Tremaine
Greg Ooi	Richard Scott	Penny Tsoutouras
Richard Osborne	Mitsuo Sekikawa	Christy Turner
Tadashi Ozaki	Tsuneo Sekimoto	Kuljeet Vaid
Tracey Parish	Kim Seow	Melanie Van Altena
Kathleen Paul	Rob Sergi	Con Vanco
Brian Penhall	Tarciso Sindeaux	Juha Varrela
Liu Ping	Patricia Smith	John Wetherell
Pertti Pirttiniemi	Richard Smith	Ted Wild
Ron Presswood	Lyndall Smythe	Grace Wong
Kris Anne Pulanco	John Spencer	Sabrina Woodroffe
Josephine Quinn	Sue Springbett	Hiroyuki Yamada
Jonathan Race	Lauren Stow	Xiaoyan Zhou
Quentin Rahaus	Smitha Sukumar	Peter Zilm
David Richmond	Sue Taji	
Jackie Rovensky	Masami Takahashi	

Adelaide Dental School staff and students
Australian Multiple Birth Association staff
Australian NHMRC Twin Registry staff
Colgate Australian Clinical Dental Research Centre staff
Colgate Oral Care Australia staff
Dental Health Services Victoria
Institute for Medical and Veterinary Science staff
Melbourne Dental School staff and students
Royal Dental Hospital of Melbourne staff
School of Dental Therapy Melbourne staff
South Australian Dental Service
Sydney Dental School staff and students
Western Sydney Local Health District
Westmead Centre for Oral Health staff
Women's and Children's Hospital Adelaide staff

Twin Studies

A GALLERY OF RESEARCHERS, TWINS AND THEIR FAMILIES

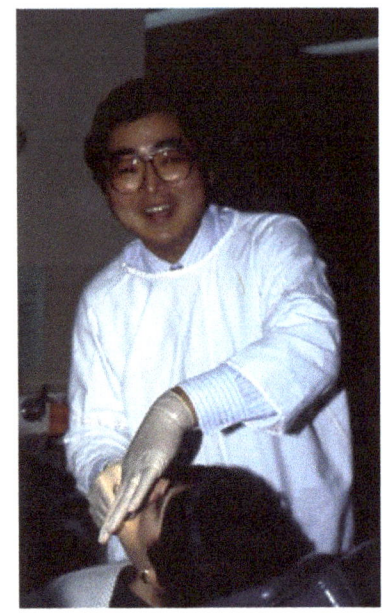
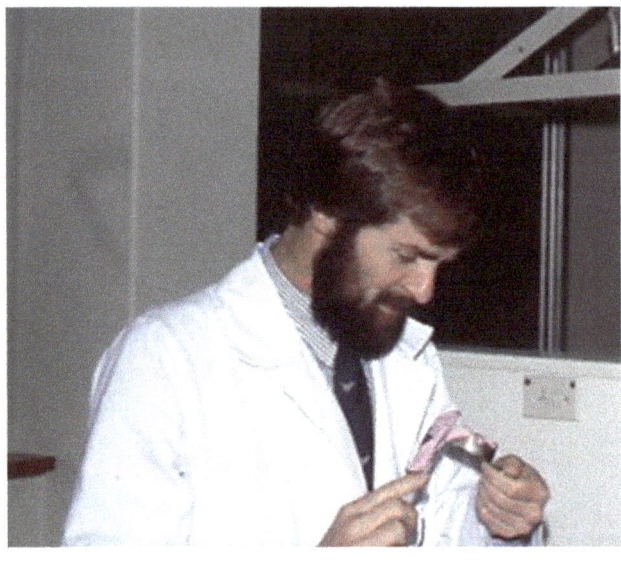
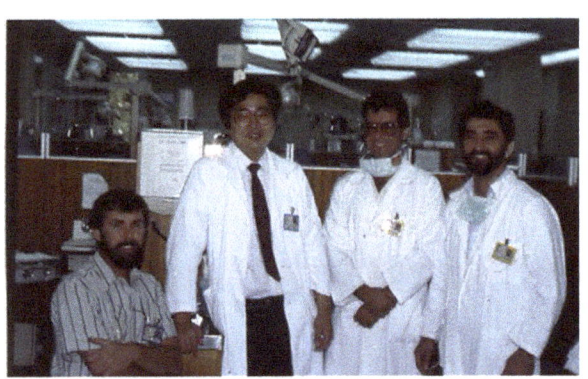
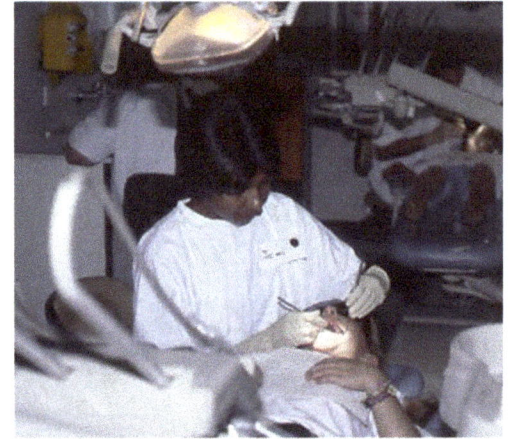
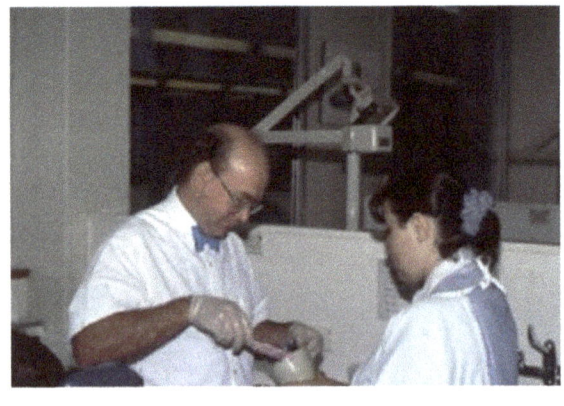
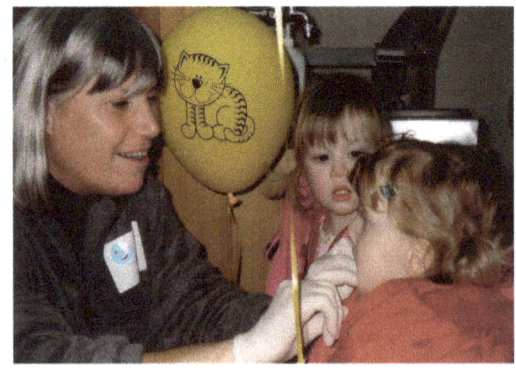

Appendix 1

Thank you Michelle for our tooth brushes & tooth paste

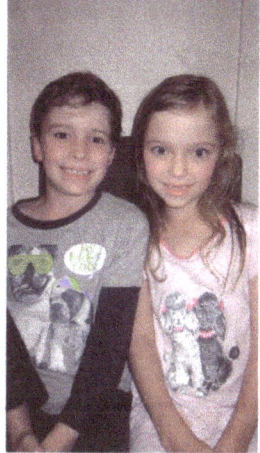
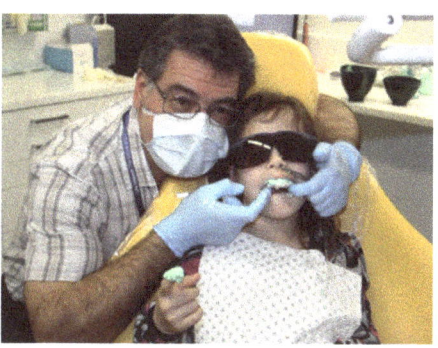
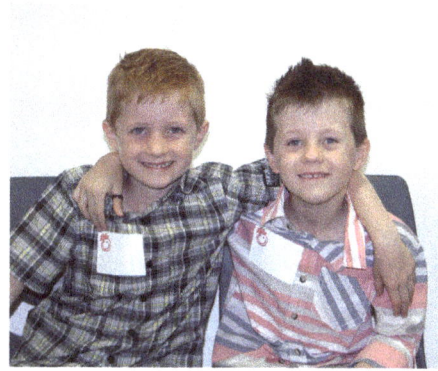
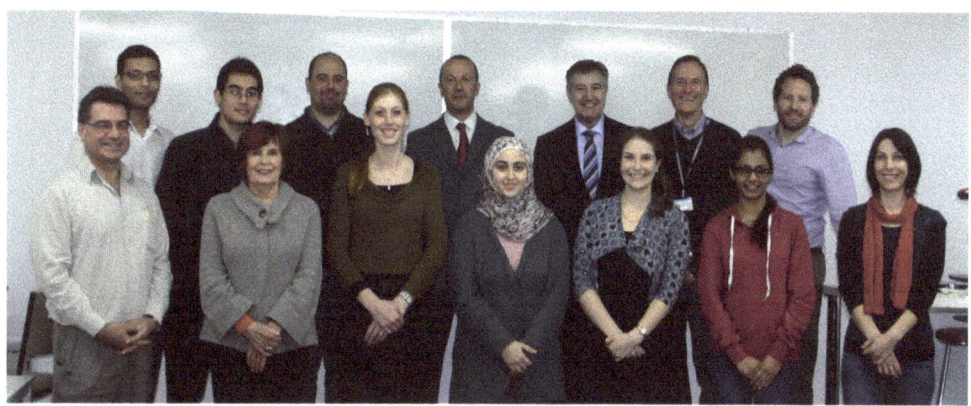
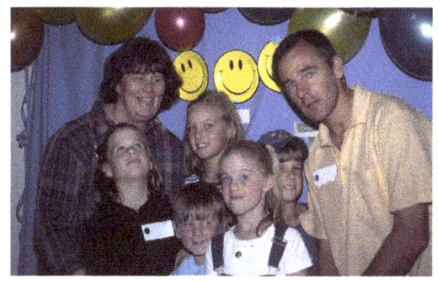
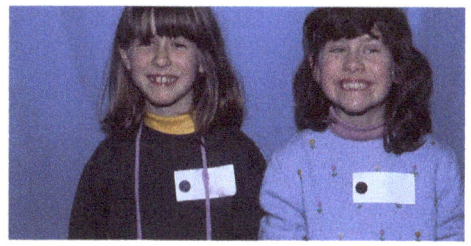

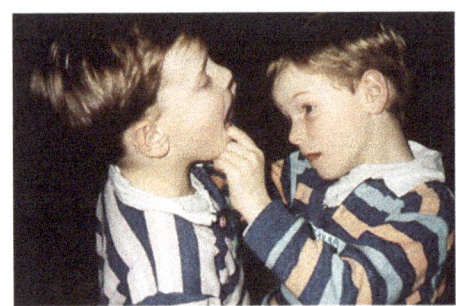
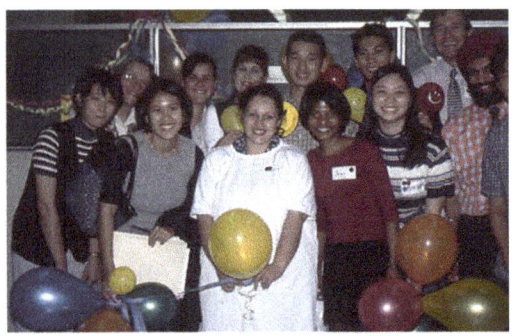
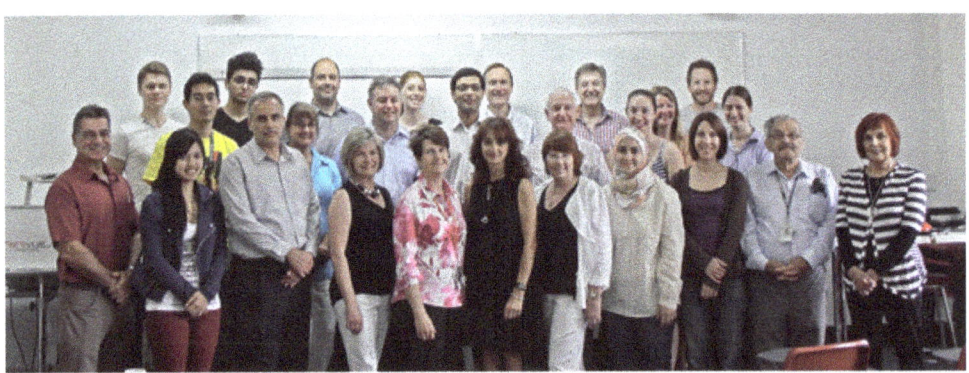
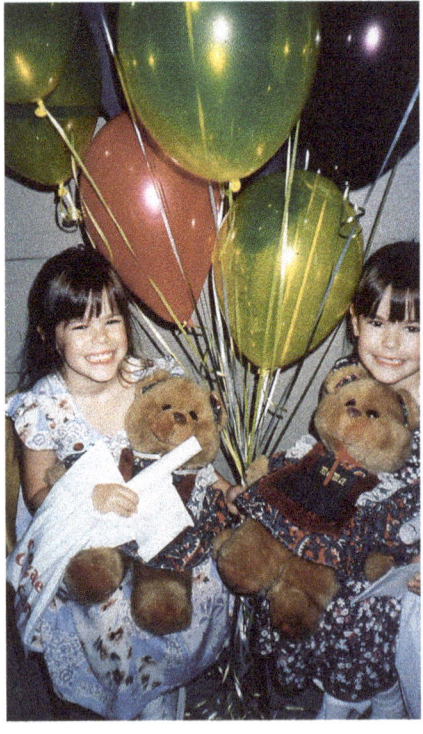
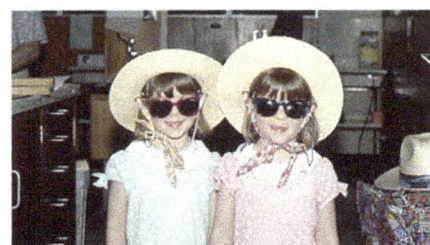
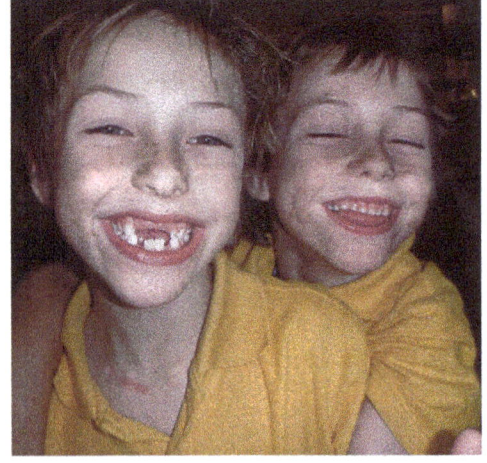

Appendix 1

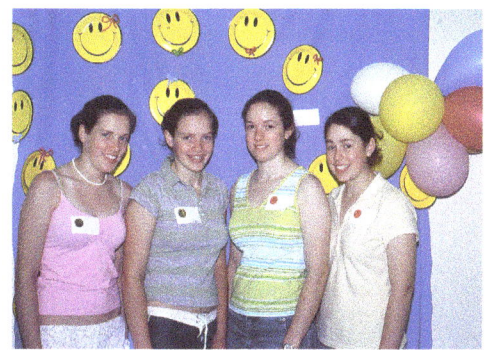
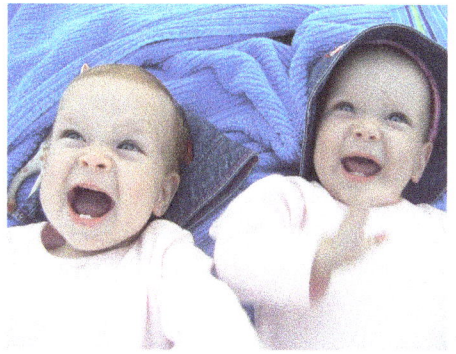
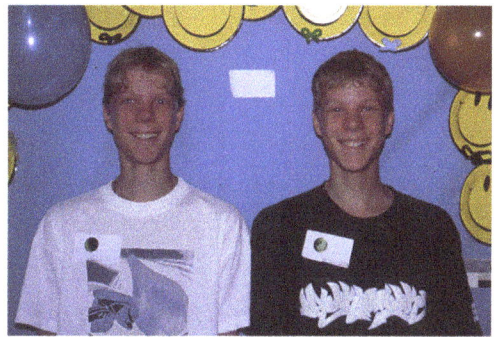
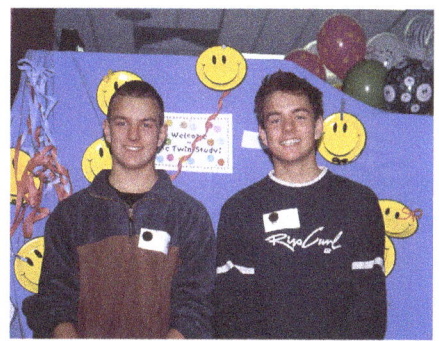
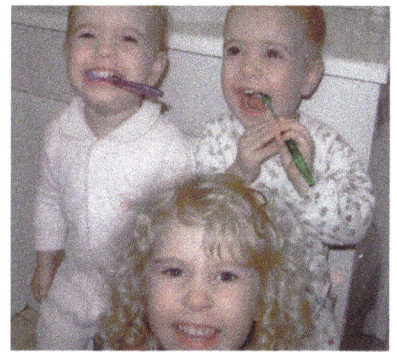
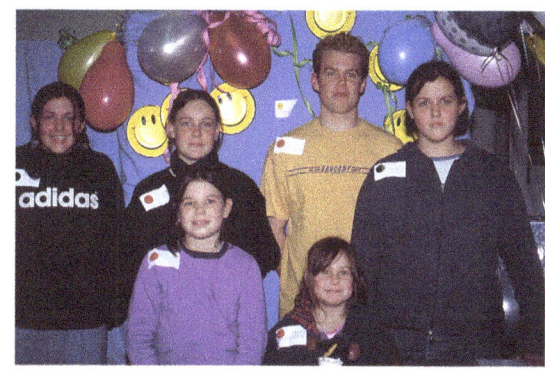
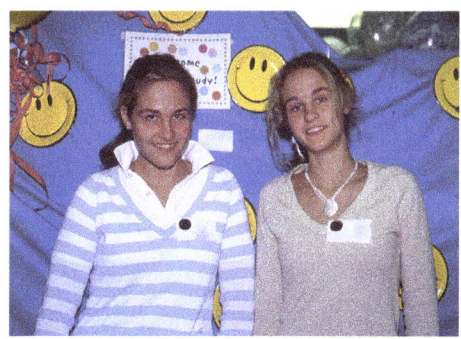
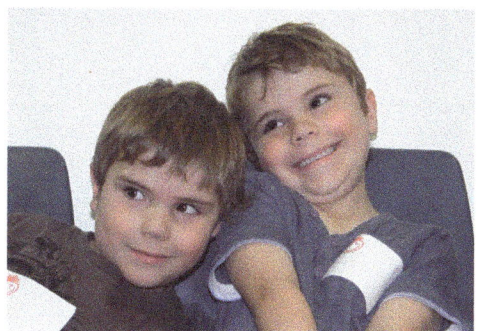

Twin Studies

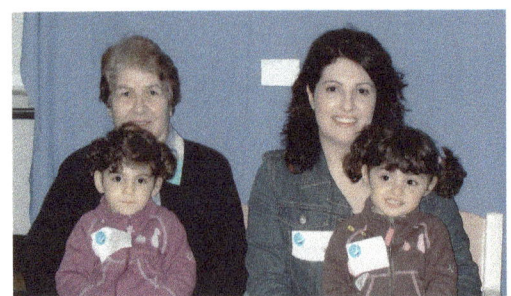
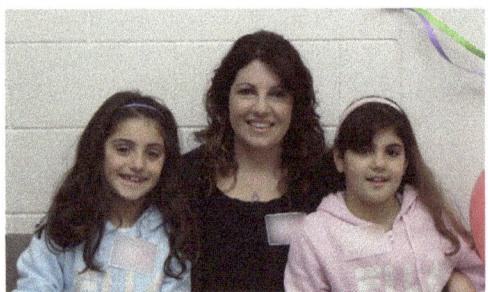
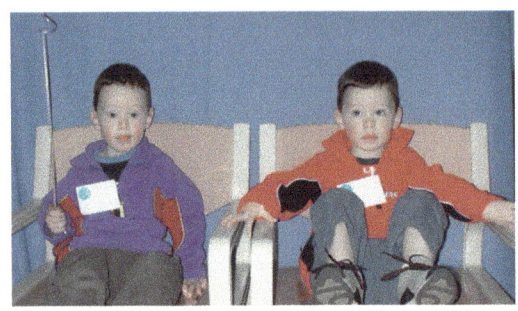
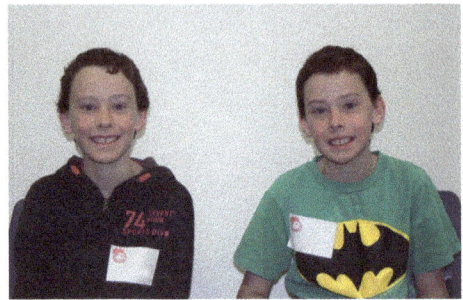
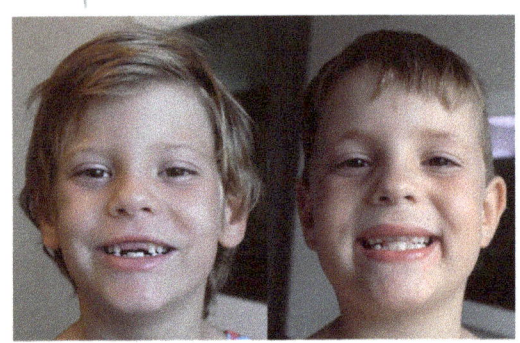
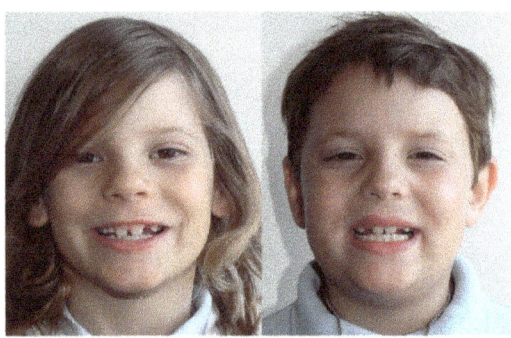
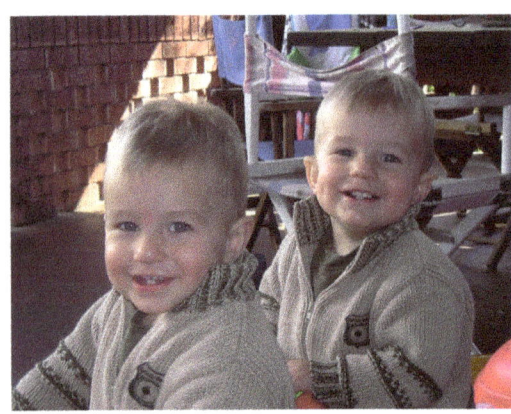
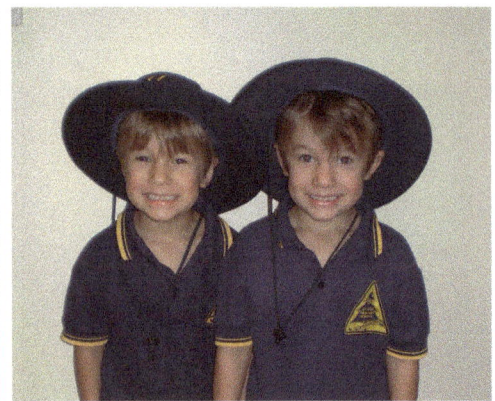

Appendix 1

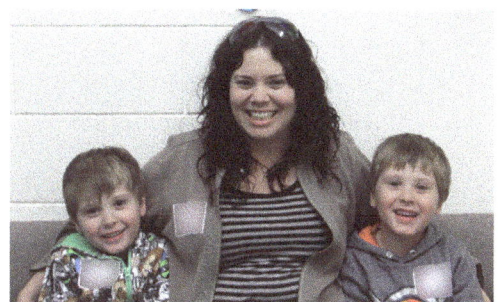
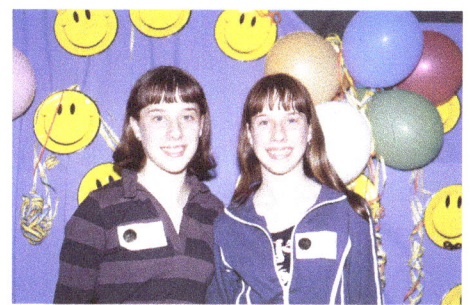
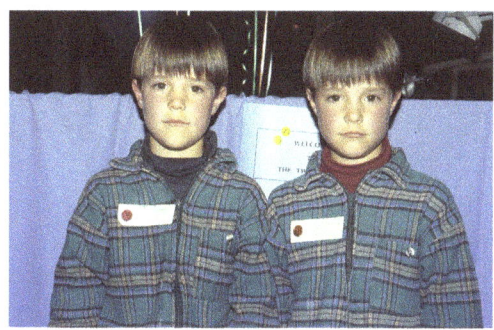
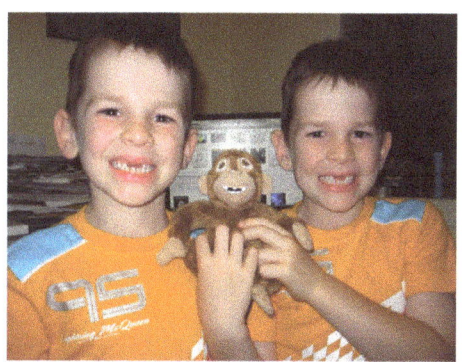
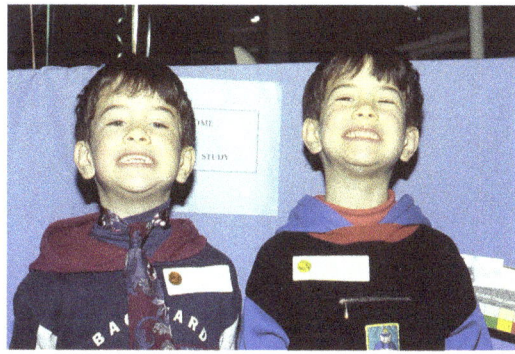
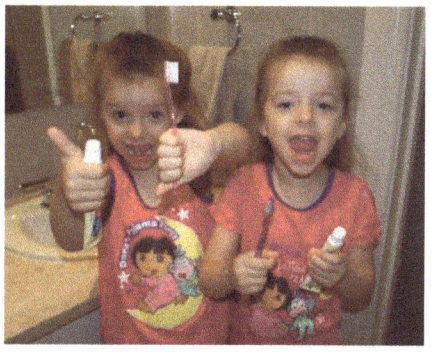
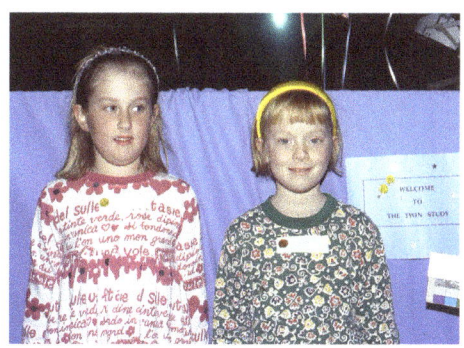
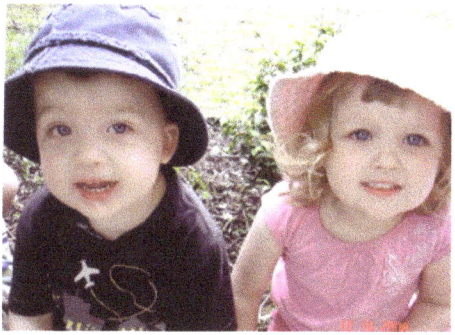

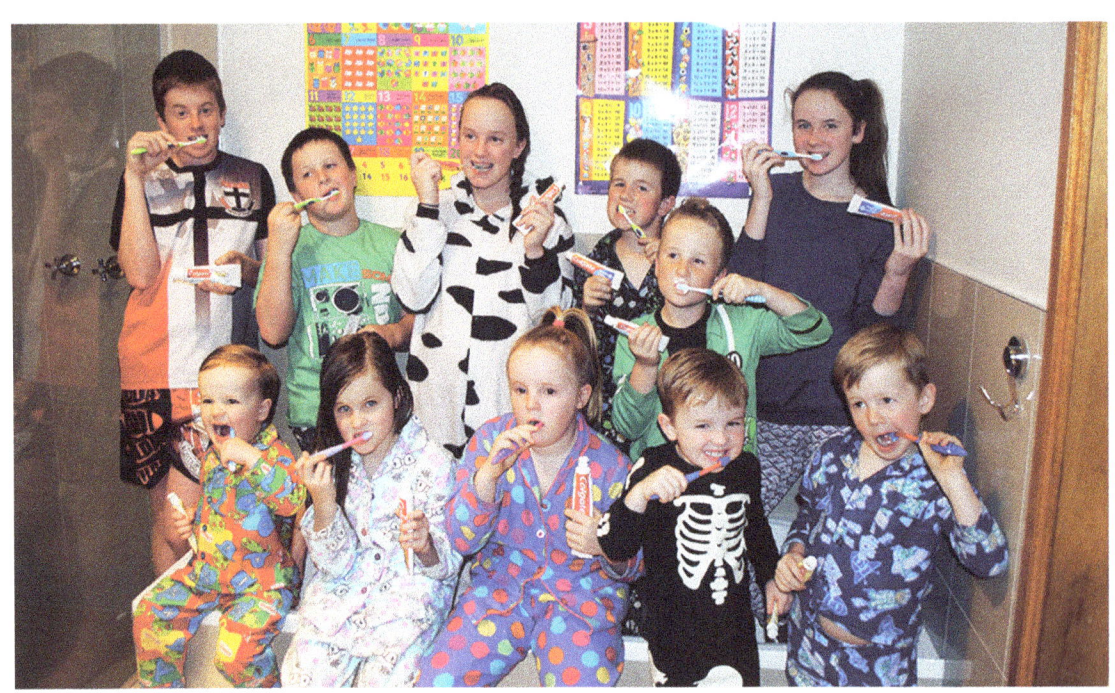

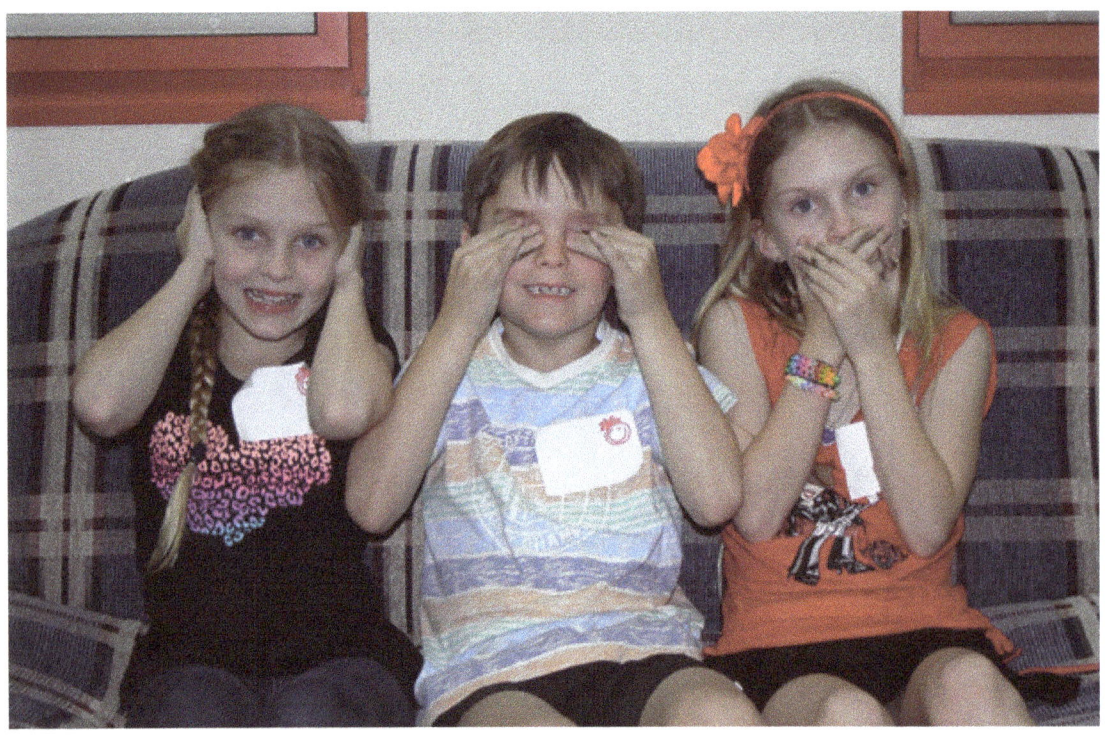

Appendix 1

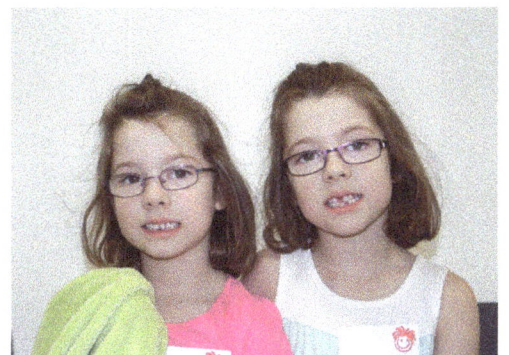
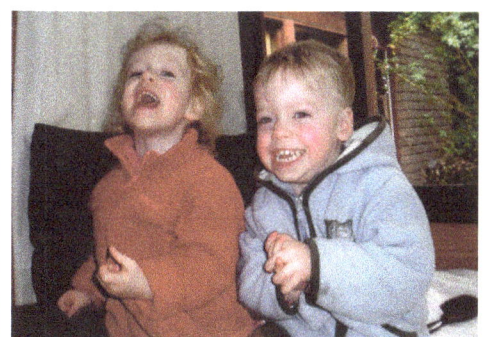
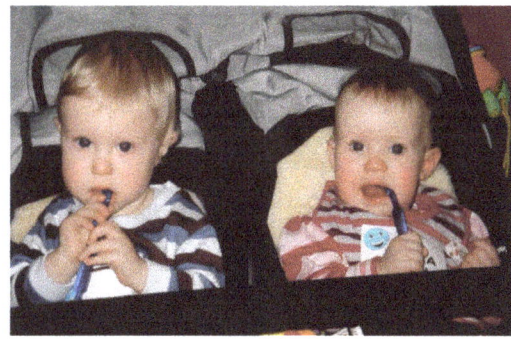
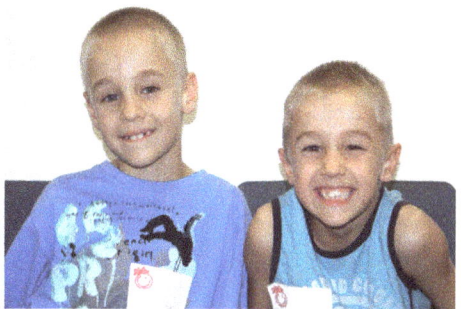
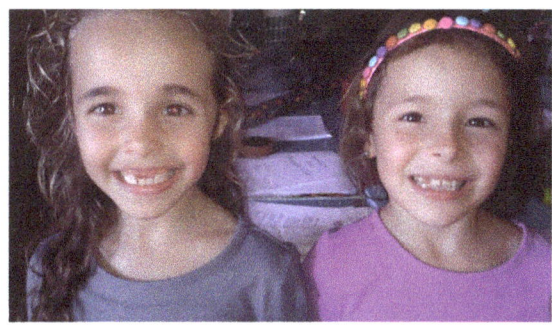
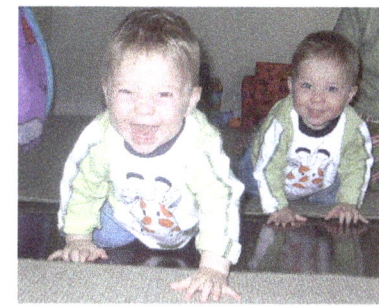
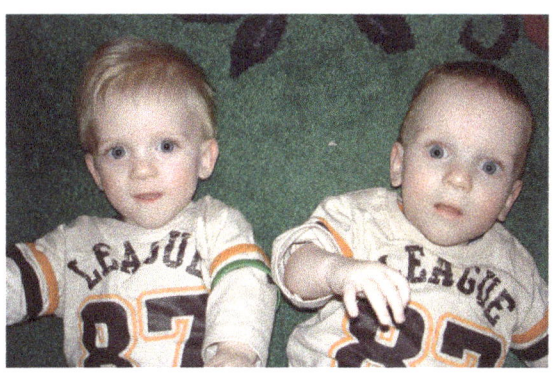
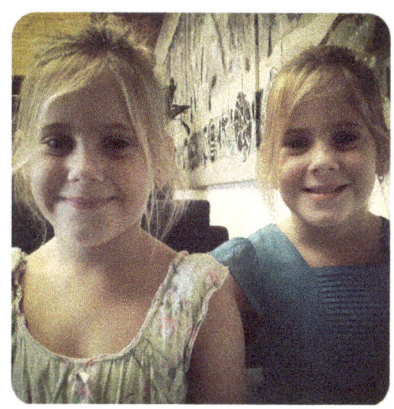

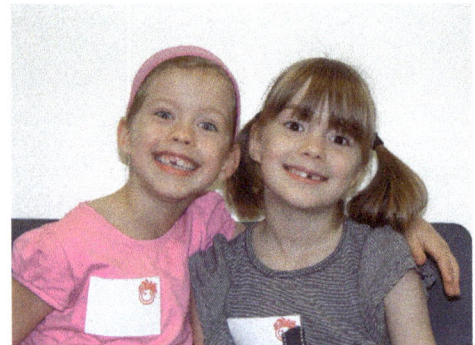
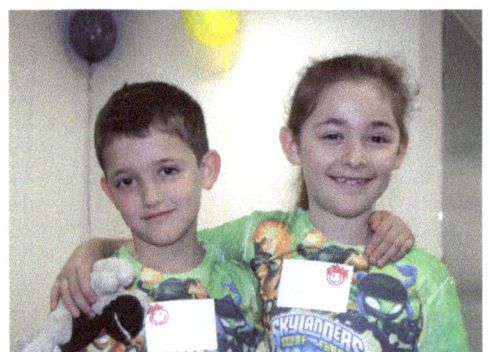
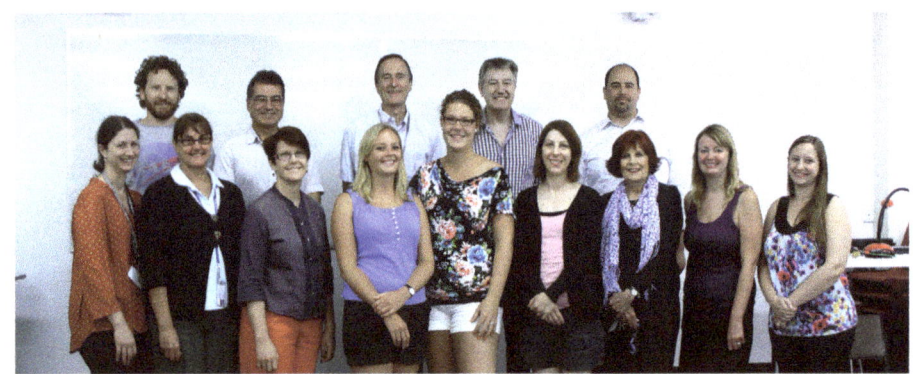
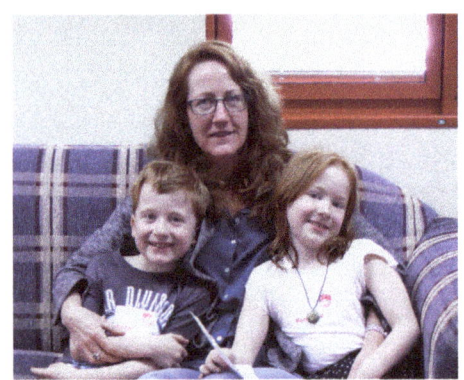
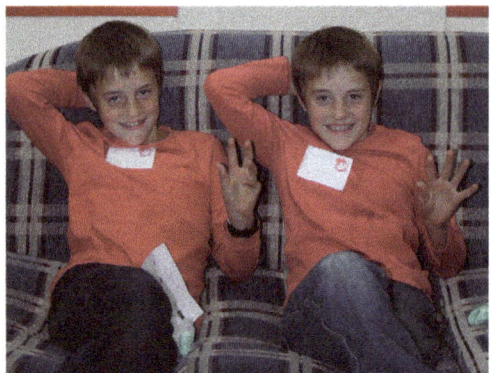
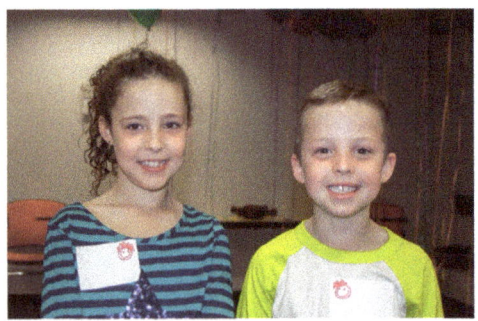
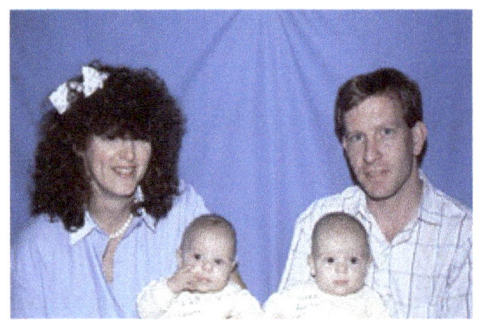

Appendix 1

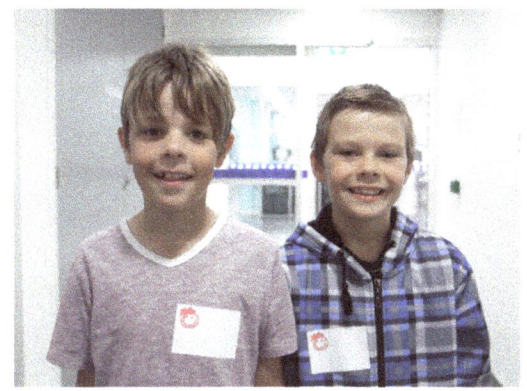
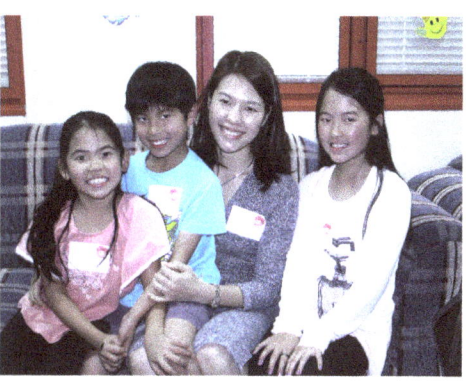
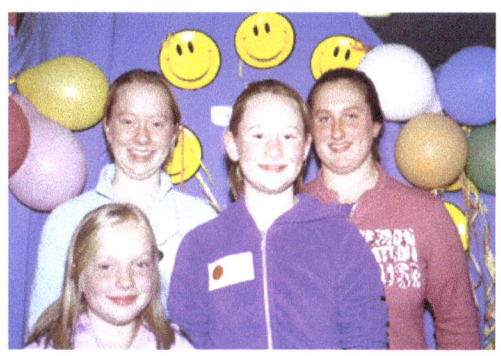
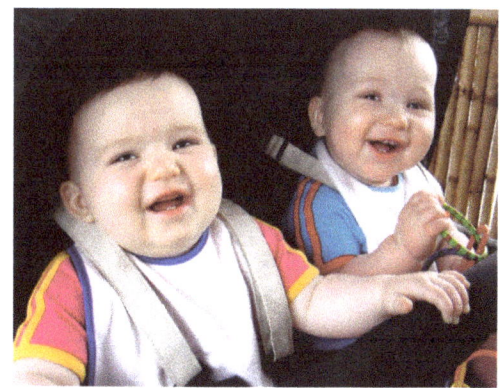
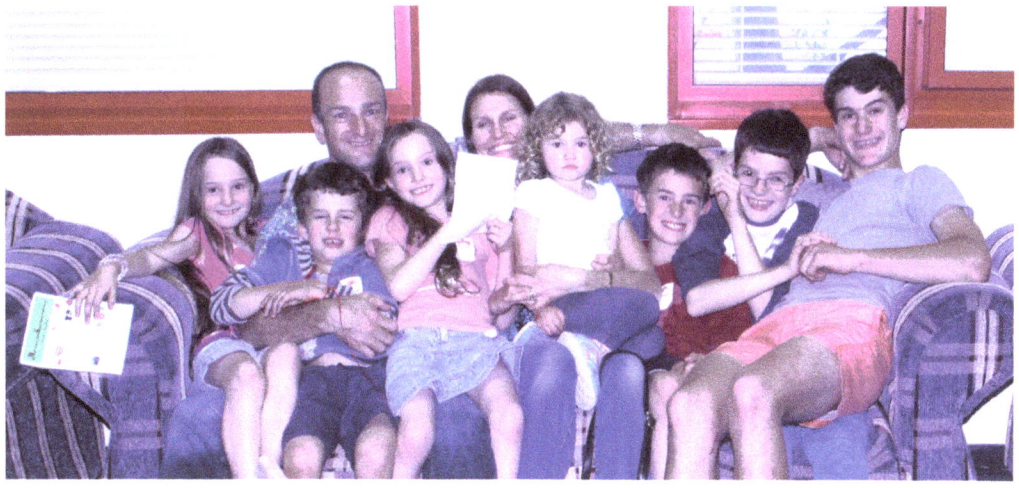

Twin Studies

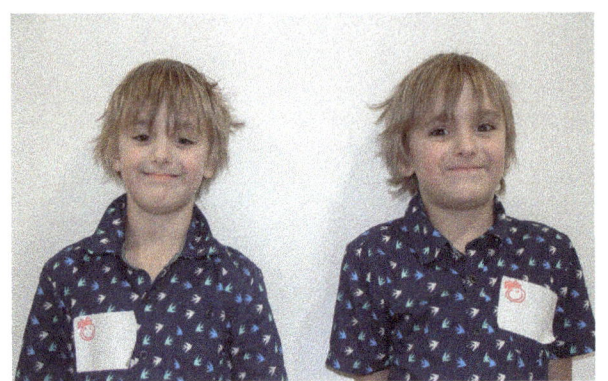
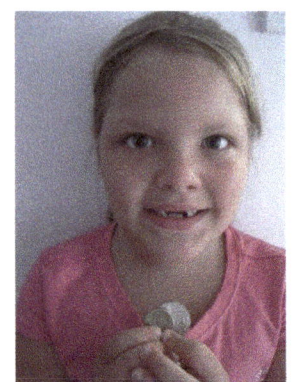
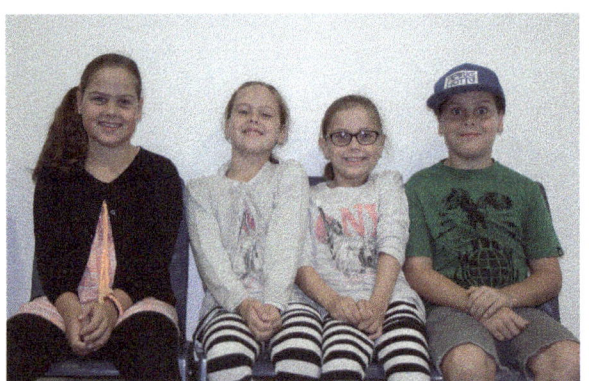
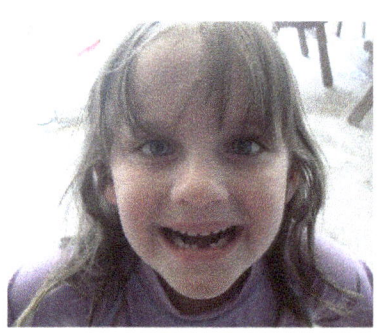
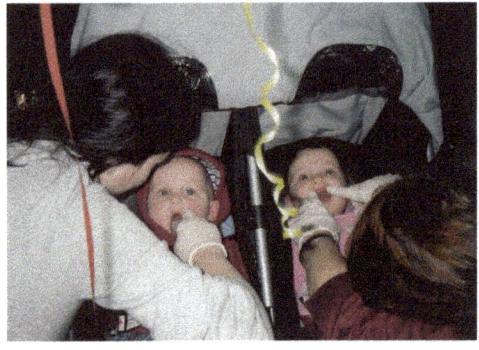
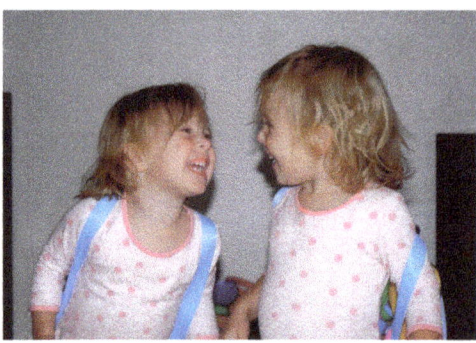
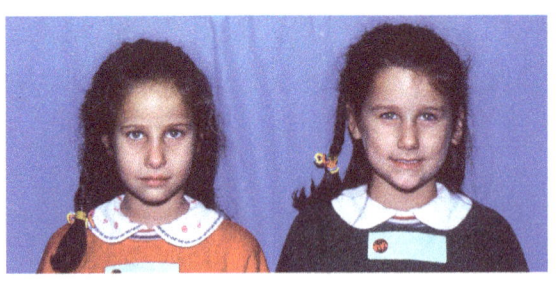
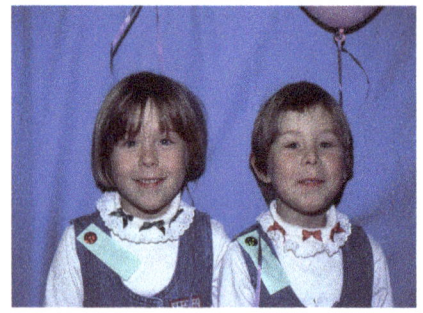

Appendix 1

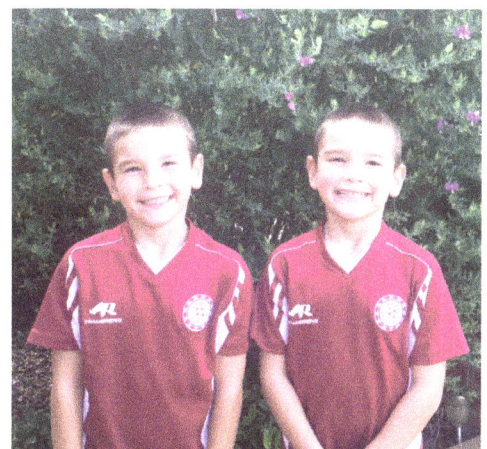
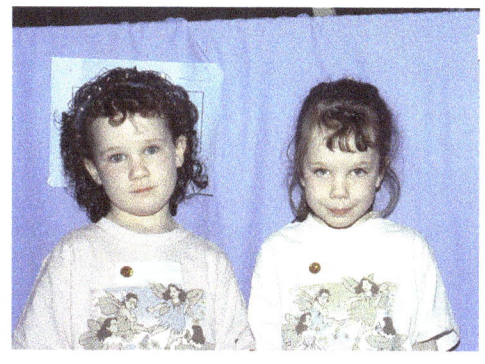
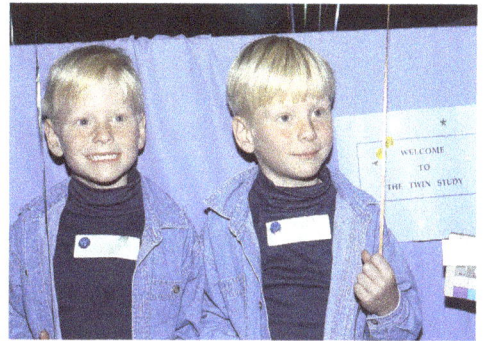
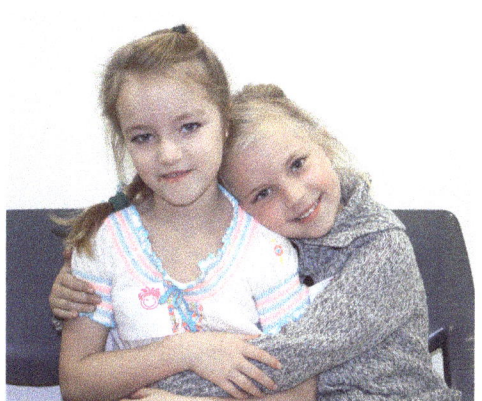
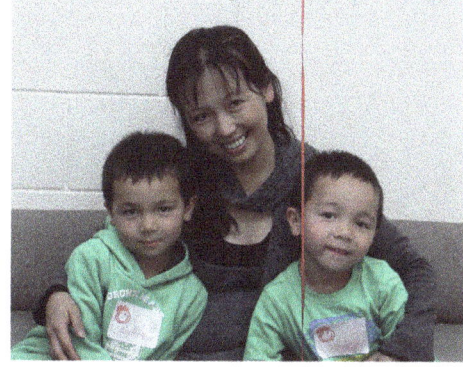
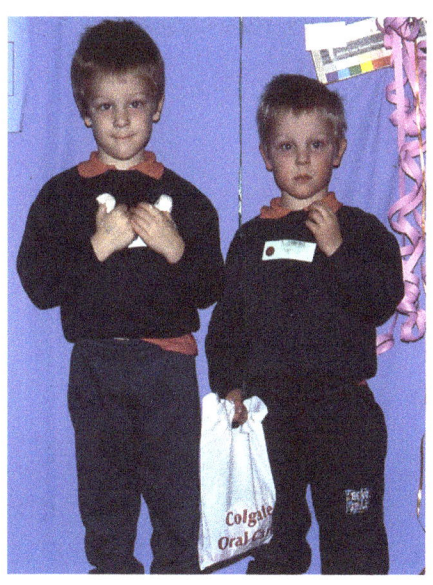
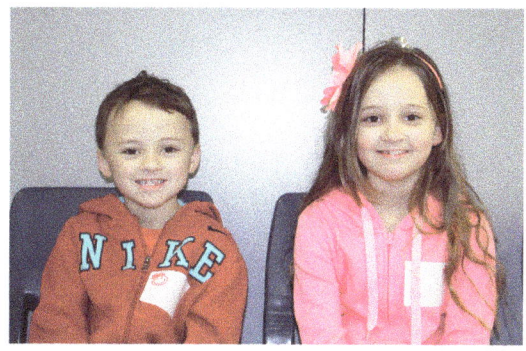

This book is available as a free fully-searchable ebook from
www.adelaide.edu.au/press

www.ingramcontent.com/pod-product-compliance
Lightning Source LLC
Chambersburg PA
CBHW040222040426
42333CB00051B/3313